THE OBESITY MYTH:

YOU'RE NOT OVERWEIGHT

YOU'RE OVERWASTE

To Ethel
1/12/2020

Life is joyous & beautiful
when lived in harmony
with nature. Flow in
harmony, live in joy

THE OBESITY MYTH:

YOU'RE NOT OVERWEIGHT

YOU'RE OVERWASTE

Aaron Mottley, CHHC

Breathe

Eat

Move

(Publishing, ISBN number and other pertinent information)

ISBN 978-0-557-68911-8

A trademark search has been conducted on the following terms and are herby claimed by the author; Biodynamic Nutrition™, Breath Mastery Technique™, Breath of Life Clinic™, Couch Fitness™, Internal Fitness Series™, LIVE~IT ™, The Art of Snacking™, and. ™ may not appear every time these terms are used throughout the book as the terms are used numerously.

Cover design by Kebo Logo and Designs at
KeboLogoDesigns.com.   Photographs for Internal Fitness Series taken by Folami Irby-Mottley

DISCLAIMER

The information in this book is the result of research, training and practices of the author. The content of this book is not intended to substitute for the professional advice or care of a physician or other health care professional. In using the techniques described you are doing so at your own risk. The author and publisher assume no responsibility or liability for any adverse conditions or effects allegedly arising from the application of any information in this book. The information in this book is not intended to prevent, treat, or cure any disease, or condition.

Dedication

I feel honored, and privileged to be able to share my insights with you. I know in my heart that you will use the following information to improve your health and well-being, and that of your family and community. When my mother died of cancer in 1989 I was profoundly impacted. She was physically and in many ways emotionally the most powerful woman I have ever known. It made no sense to me for someone so strong and seemingly unshakable to have to suffer so and leave so untimely. She possessed an inner wisdom and unwavering desire to help others. Many endeavors throughout my life have been undertaken with her watching over, whether physically present or not. I have and will always reflect on my actions and think, will this make her proud, or disappointed, knowing I could do better. This is one of those times that I feel her smile of pride and approval. Yep, I think I've done Mrs. Massie Lee (NancyLee), and Mr. Edgar proud.

A special thanks to Shelley and Karen, the mothers of my four beautiful children: Arán, Kian, Folami, and Jahi. And a gracious thank you to them for choosing me to be their Father in this lifetime, I pray that I never disappoint you.

Preface

Being obese or overweight is merely a symptom of a far greater problem. A problem that is common to many besides the overweight or obese. Modern science has conditioned us to attack symptoms and not the problem. We have become blinded to observing what is symptom versus what is problem. When treating a symptom and not the problem you create a myriad of side affects and leave the problem to run its course. The problem here is the accumulation of waste and toxins in the body. Its eventual natural outcome is the deterioration of the body, beginning with the break down of its organs and systems. This breakdown in its many forms and presentation is what we call disease. The obvious answer is to prevent or stop the accumulation of waste and toxins, and remove what has already accumulated. That is the focus of the information in this book.

The mandatory disclaimer designed to protect those who write anecdotal quote "non-scientific information," is exact. The information presented is indeed not intended to prevent, treat or cure any disease or condition. The body will do that all on its own once the waste and toxins are removed. This three book series is presented as one book because it is a three part answer to the issues of the day. Each subject deserves to be written as an individual book in it's own right. Which is why this is written as a compilation. As a whole they comprise the solution at the core of what plagues man in this time. What is so amazing about the information presented here is that each bit of information is very simple on its own. You have already heard a lot of what is presented here. The improvement is in how the information is presented. As you integrate the many simple bits and pieces into your life you will love the simplicity. You will also appreciate the way your life and the lives of your loved ones will be transformed.

This overall book is presented as a compilation of three books born of trinity of principles. These principles separately comprise a book of their own but the trinity combines to create the essence of properly maintaining the human form. The principles **O. N. E.** are **O**xygen: presented in the Breath Mastery book; **N**utrition: presented in the Biodynamic Nutrition book; and **E**xercise presented in the Internal Fitness Series book.

BOOK

ONE

BREATH

MASTERY

Breath Mastery

Table of Contents

Introduction

Book One of the Trinity

Oxygen   Nutrition   Exercise

This body of work came about after I asked several questions dealing with the current state of health. Especially in the America and more importantly, that of women and children. My desire was to come up with simple straightforward solutions that could be implemented with ease. Implemented in a way that would not take you out of your regular day-to-day life. Though these changes are simple and concise they will bring about a change in lifestyle for many.

The primary question I asked of the universe was, "What is the most effective and efficient way to deal with the issues of hypertension, heart dis-ease, diabetes, obesity, arthritis, cancer the many forms of dis-ease that have become the plagues of modern day life?" The answer I got was, rid the body of toxins. Simple enough, right? Then of course I had to ask, "How do you do that?" That answer came just as simple. Go to the waste line spelled waistline for you fashionable people, and empty it of waste, perpetually. Then of course another how do you do that question, you can see where this going, right? To make a long story short, I was given the **O. N. E.** answer I was looking for.

While getting the answers to these questions not only did I do thorough analysis of the physical body I wound up going on an unforeseen journey. Over the last two decades plus I have studied: Herbology, Chi Gong, Kemetic Yoga, something that was not even present in my awareness beforehand and taken a Holistic Health Consultant certification course. The latter course allowed me to be temporarily registered as a Naturopathic Doctor. More stuff I hadn't anticipated. During this journey my body was transformed as I continued personal research for my own edification and enlightenment.

I began my study of the breath some years ago, rather impractically and guided by unexpected influences. The most pronounced was nearly two decades ago, while reading a magazine article about Free Divers. Those phenomenally adventurous souls who dive to great depths in the ocean unaided by air tanks. The feat of holding ones breath for extended periods beyond the average let alone doing so down to depths of a hundred feet or more was captivating. Needless to say I wanted to try. The holding my breath part, not the diving part. The article described the unusual techniques this particular diver had developed to increase lung capacity and the oxygenation of the blood.

Some years later I took a short course in the Six Healing sounds as practiced by Chi Gong practitioners. My instructor was Peggy Li at the Song Ho Health Center in Silver Spring, Maryland. The idea of using the breath and sound vibrations created within the body to stimulate energy flow into the organs. This too I found to be very profound. Then in the last few years Kemetic Yoga and a revisiting of the Six Healing sounds. Except, this time as taught by a Taoist practitioner. Promptly following that was the Certified Holistic Health Consultant course.

Throughout the years I would stretch a bit to keep my body loose and relaxed. But fully immersing into, and becoming certified to teach a form of Yoga was definitely unanticipated. Something I now thoroughly appreciate. The breath is key and tied to the movement intricately in Kemetic Yoga. I first learned the Cleansing Breath. This was an awakening. By the way my teacher and mentor was Master Yersir Ra Hotep. I continued my study for a time with Master Kwesi Karamoko, who instructs on Ausaurian Tantric Yoga, a form of Kemetic Yoga. Through Yersir I was also introduced to Dr. Wayne B. Chandler, author of Ancient Future: The Teachings and Prophetic Wisdom of the Seven Hermetic Laws of Ancient Egypt. He is the aforementioned Taoist practitioner. Dr. Chandler also instructed on Tongue Positioning another Taoist practice that attunes ones energies.

After practicing both the Cleansing Breath and Tongue Positioning I began to combine the two and found a great reward that I call the Breath Mastery Technique™. This technique is the core of the Breath Mastery book and a newfound awareness that transforms and reenergizes the body, mind and spirit. It further aids in the accelerated ridding the body of waste and toxins. The Breath of Life Clinic™ applies this technique alternating with the Breath of Fire technique. I created this short but very dynamic series to affect an intense form of interval training. This expedites the changing of the breathing pattern and greater uptake of oxygen. Which dramatically increases the metabolism, quickly builds stamina, burns fat and facilitates better digestion.

I have been studying and seeking for years. Looking for the most effective, concise, and easily adaptable means to maintain the human form and prepare if for transcendence. Though it is not the same journey, in principle, I liken it to that of Bruce Lee. He sought the ultimate form of undefeatable martial art. He studied many styles and with many masters. After a time a certain awareness crystallized in his mind. The answer he sought was not in the movement and forms he and many others studied, but in the principles used to create them. Analyzing these principles and adapting them, he would strip down the movements. Down to bare essentials and reorganize them to come up with a form without form. A martial art that was adaptive to the individual and his or her individual attributes. I too know now that in order to master anything you must first master the very basic principles of that thing. I believe as I have analyzed various principles surrounding health and wellness that the **O. N. E.** methodology is on that same scale. I welcome all who are looking for a better life, unencumbered by the burdens of toxic buildup in the body. I don't proclaim to be a healer; in my opinion only those who can project their energy into the body of another and transform their health are true healers. Outside of that the body heals itself. We only need give it what it needs for that purpose. Now let us take up this journey together to do just that.

Chapter 1

The Breath of Life

Genesis 2:7: And the Lord God formed man of the dust of the ground, and breathed into his nostrils the breath of life; and man became a living soul.

The Holy Bible; King James Version.

Chi is life force energy and is all around us and in everything. When we breathe in we breathe in Chi.

It is scientific fact that we cannot live but for only a short period without oxygen.

> **No matter which belief system(s) you have there is a simple constant; if you breathe; *it is,* THE BREATH OF LIFE.**

There is much debate about when life actually begins, at the point of conception, a certain stage of fetal growth? While this is an ongoing debate there is no dispute that once we are born the most crucial point of life is immediate. We must begin to breathe. From that moment on the breath is the essence of life itself. Life outside of the womb begins with the first breath, and until we take our last breath, we are alive.

With this simple and basic premise we can see how important breathing is and why it shouldn't be taken lightly. Yet, for the majority, that is just what we do. Like many things in life, until we face the possibility of loosing it we take it for granted. In our unaware and unconscious moving through our day-to-day lives we lose awareness of how vital the breath is and it's power. This life force energy that we take for granted is truly wondrous and magical. *Think about it, simply breathing allows us to have a soul, a mind, a body and all the complex and magical things that come along with being alive.* Something that powerful should never be taken for granted. It needs to be cultivated, honored and respected. For then we can begin to appreciate it, and harness its true power. The most basic component of life, it's beginning and end. We can begin living a life of mastery by mastering life on it most basic and simple terms. Mastery of the breath is the beginning of the mastery of life. As with the mastery of anything there are many levels one can achieve. Also as with the mastery of anything you must first master the basics. Which always begins with the first lesson and principle. In this case it is the Breath.

So in this series what you will witness, experience and achieve with application, is the beginning of and/or continuation of life mastery. This work is foundational. Many of our lives are built on faulty foundations. Foundations that have lead to many unfortunate situations. This foundation work can correct many of these situations at their very core. Whether physical, emotional, mental or spiritual, all can be affected by going back and shoring up this pillar of life's foundation.

On a physical level increasing the amount of oxygen and lowering the carbon dioxide levels in the blood, revitalizes the entire body. It increases energy and vitality and balances the body's alkalinity and acidity. On an emotional level it calms and relieves anxiety, circumvents anger, and elevates our mood. On a mental level it increases clarity. On a spiritual level it strengthens our ability to be more loving, accepting, and forgiving. It creates a spiraling synergy that continues with practice and time. All of the above mentioned influences lend themselves to lower blood pressure through less constriction and inflammation in and around the blood vessels. Instantly and with continued practice we arrive at greater levels of relaxation and meditation. This leads to greater focus and creativity, greater abilities, and contributions to our lives and the lives of those around us. Like life itself the possibilities of our abilities and achievements don't end until we take that last *Breath of Life*.

MASTER THE BREATH AND BEGIN THE MASTERY OF LIFE.

Chapter 2

Breath Mastery Technique

We're starting this chapter by getting right into the exercise. This book is intended to inform, and give decisive tools for improvement of health and well-being. This chapter and the next will take you right into the exercises then give you a breakdown on how and why they were developed. So here we go, do the following just as described and you will experience something very dynamic. For many it will be the fullest breath you have ever taken. Before doing this exercise sit or stand as relaxed as possible and count the number of your breaths per minute. Then count the number of breaths after you're done. Make sure to write these numbers down in your Healthy Transitions Journal (see Appendix). Take note of how much deeper and longer each breath becomes. Also notice how you are simultaneously both relaxed and invigorated. Extend the exhalation as you progress. As you do this you will tone and strengthen the abdominal muscles considerably. One quick caution, don't overdo the inhalation; do not strain the lungs. Breath work should be done on an empty stomach. *It should not be done when severely constipated or during pregnancy.*

Breath Mastery Technique:

- **Place tip of the tongue to back of roof of mouth with the mouth closed.**

- **Inhale as slowly as possible through the nostrils; into abdomen then chest, feeling the air on back of the throat audibly making inhalation sound.**

- **Pause for 3 count.**

- **Release the tongue; gently relax jaw, opening mouth slightly.**

- **Exhale through mouth as slowly as possible with an audible *haah* sound, as if you were fogging up a mirror, fully express the breath.**

- **Pause for 3 count; repeat sequence for a minimum of 5 breaths**

This breathing technique cannot be overdone. The more you practice the better and healthier you will become. Consider your health and the overall benefits this will bring to your entire body as you practice. It is imperative that an increasing percentage of your breathing becomes deeper and fuller. This is an extremely passive yet very dynamic technique free of the risk of hyperventilation. You will practice it at your leisure when reading, watching TV, at the movies, at your desk, or in the car, do it often.

Continue this exercise at will while reading and throughout life. As stated in the previous chapter the breath is quintessential to life itself. Maximizing the breath several intervals during each day will dramatically change your ability to deal with stress. It will also improve your energy level, metabolism, and digestion. The best times to do any breath work are in the morning upon rising, before any meal, between bowel movements, and definitely before any form of exercise. It is perfect for beginning relaxation, massage, meditation and preparation for sleep, very beneficial before, during and after any stressful situation (anxiety). It helps couples harmonize and become more spiritually, emotionally and physically in sync. *Ever hear of being equally yoked or of one accord? Start with being of one breath.*

Upon rising:

Starting your day. While still lying in bed take a few moments to do this exercise. It will calm, and energize you. This will allow you to gather your thoughts about the day and what you want to accomplish in a peaceful and positive fashion. Many of us jump up and start running from the moment we open our eyes in the morning. Beginning our day with the notion that it's going to be hectic and overwhelming. Practice relaxing for a few moments at the very beginning of the day and fill your lungs with a breath of fresh air. Allow your mind to be calm and still, know that there is joy and fulfillment in life. Know that the positive vibrations you send out and begin the day with will be returned and fill your day.

Before eating:

When you sit down for any meal do this exercise to prepare the body for nourishment that will be both satisfying and fulfilling. Many of us eat entirely to fast. Which causes indigestion, heartburn, acid reflux, poor digestion, and constipation. My mother had a phrase she used. She would tell us that we weren't eating properly because instead of chewing all we did was, "cut and swallow." Years ago as a Barber I told this to a family, as I watched one of the pre-teen boys eat a burger. They laughed. Though it was not my intent to poke fun, for I spoke with the same concern my mother did, he briefly wound up with the nickname; Cut n Swallow.

After taking a few moments to relax, the first bite should be savored. *Savoring is a lost art that only the most fervent chocolate lovers seem to really master.* I mean think about it. Food should be a culinary delight, even if it's just a piece of celery. When we appreciate food more it does the same for us. Savoring stimulates saliva, filled with enzymes; part of the first stage of digestion. When we are relaxed and savor our food it allows us to begin the chewing process with patience and appreciation. The longer we savor the first few bites the more stimulated the saliva glands are. If we are relaxed when we chew our food we take our time and mix in enough saliva that we don't find ourselves having to drink while we are eating. To quote *"wash our food down."* If you have to wash the food down basically you haven't chewed it enough as you are probably trying to swallow chunks. In this case there is not enough saliva to lubricate the lining of the throat as the foods attempts to slide through. This is problematic as the water dilutes the already inadequate amount of digestive fluid. Compounding to extend the time of digestion making the body and metabolism sluggish, creating constipation. Food that doesn't get digested in a timely fashion often winds up getting stored as fat.

Between bowel movements:

Let me make sure I'm not misleading here. Breathing exercises should facilitate movement of the bowels. DO NOT, I repeat DO NOT, do the exercises if you already feel a need to go. DO NOT do these exercises if you are severely constipated, and most definitely if you are PREGNANT.

When we fully engage the breath between eliminations it not only relaxes us it also makes for a more productive following movement. I have been told by others, *to their surprise, not mine*, that it helped to relieve constipation. This can be simply explained by the fact that the excretory organs get a gentle but dynamic massage. This massage increases their function by waking them up and squeezing more out of them. They are also more invigorated by the increased oxygen. Also, when you gently extend the exhalation as in this exercise it tightens the abdominal wall to further the massage. While I'm at it let me talk about positioning for a moment.

PROCESS OF ELIMINATION: *Get yourself a footstool and place it in front of the toilet. Place your feet on the stool. Make sure that when your feet are in place the bend in the back of the knee is above the bend in the front of the hip. This puts the body in the natural position intended for elimination. We are designed to go while squatting.* This not only puts added pressure on the abdomen it also curves the sigmoid colon, bringing it into the natural alignment necessary for a fully productive movement. Think of it this way. If you have several small trash baskets throughout your house, when it's time to take out the trash you don't empty a portion of them. Instead you empty them all. Imagine your house over time if you constantly let a portion of the trash accumulate. It would become unlivable and putrid. If you don't fully empty the intestines of what's ready to be released every time, you're allowing waste and toxins to accumulate. Which over time can have dire results. The breath and proper positioning are the beginning and end of a high quality waste removal system.

Before exercising:

Often before beginning any exercise or physical activity we are told that it is very good to warm up first. This is great advice. I would like to add to that by saying, do this breath technique also. The Breath of Life Clinic is an even better warm up exercise. This relieves a lot of tension and anxiety that one may have before an event. Speaking of events, this will do the same before any performance or appearance before an audience. Along with releasing anxiety it also oxygenates the blood. When engaged in extensive physical activity the muscles use up a lot of oxygen. Those with greater oxygen stores and greater lungpower have greater stamina. Any athlete or fan can tell you. It's not a pretty thing when you run out of gas before the end of the game or reaching the finish line. A lot of boxers lose because they ran out of gas. As I mentioned in the introduction free divers perform extensive breathing exercises before diving. Using advanced techniques to hyper oxygenate their blood and extend their breath. You don't have to be a world-class athlete or extreme sportsperson to benefit from increased oxygen intake. They do however give us great examples of our true potential.

> Get yourself a footstool. When seated on the toilet make sure that the bend in the back of the knee is higher than the bend in the front of the hip.

Preparation for relaxation, sleep or meditation and stress management:

This is the easy one. When teaching the Breath Mastery Technique I'm always amazed at how many people actually wind up yawning by the third breath. I'm confident many of you upon your first attempt will wind up doing the same. Many of us have a hard time relaxing. Often nights are filled with restlessness. Slowing the breath and filling the lungs allows for full relaxation. Filling the lower portion of the lungs with good clean oxygen and ridding it of stale carbon dioxide that may not get expelled on a regular basis accomplishes this. Similar to the previous example of fully taking out all of the trash. If you've done Yoga, Tai Chi, Chi Gong, meditation or hypnosis, you are aware of the power of the breath, and it's ability to facilitate relaxation. In Yoga using the breath allows us to relax and extend our movement and ability to get into postures that we wouldn't be able to otherwise. In Tai Chi and Chi Gong the breath aids the fluidity of movement. In meditation and hypnosis it allows us to transcend our conscious mind and tap into the power of the subconscious.

Learning to control the breath enables us to begin our journey anew. Our journey of transcendence: transcending pain, toxic emotions, toxic waste in the body and all the issues that accompany them. I have had a cavity filled without any anesthesia because I employed deep, slow, rhythmic breathing. I have and will often state that in order to master anything you must first master the basics of that particular thing. The mastery of life begins with mastering its most basic and powerful component, the breath. I've heard that when you pray you talk to God, and that when you meditate you listen to God. I believe this because when you are in deep meditation you are at a place of serenity where only God can be heard.

Building healthier relationships:

When you examine the benefits detailed in this book of the Breath Mastery Technique there is a realization that you are made healthier and more whole. Better prepared for a more fulfilled life, creating a healthier and better you to offer the world and your partner. When practiced on a regular basis as a couple you can arrive at a Oneness of Spirit. Practicing the BMT and the Breath of Life Clinic together will also help bring greater harmony to your relationship. This will allow for growth and harmony in the general community, helping to create a better world. Think about it. All this good health and Internal Fitness, along with more harmonious relationships will make the world a better place. These simple practices are foundational and transformative. When implemented on a local, national scale and beyond we can all move into a space toward greater human development.

Couples that have longevity on their side will tell you that it takes a lot of work and staying focused. Adding the practices herein will lend to making that work a lot easier. It will also ensure that even those couples will have greater love and even longer lasting healthier relationships. Plus there will be more of them. For creating greater harmony, health and vibrancy in a relationship truly is Making Love. Many consider the physical act of sexual intercourse as Making Love. Making Love is really spiritual and has a deeper more profound meaning.

Making: verb: the act of creating.

Love: noun: a state of being that encompasses the deepest care, respect and honor.

When in a relationship and your actions toward your partner are sincere and of this nature, *you are Making Love.* I've often heard that people should have more SEX. While I agree with this statement it should be expanded. People in relationships should have healthier more responsible and nurturing SEX. In Tantric SEX, couples start out by breathing together. They do this while either back to back or in an embrace. After a brief period their breath, heartbeats, and energies synchronize. This allows for harmonious flow and movement. Flowing rhythmically, slowing the pace, pausing and being mindful of the breath, deeply gazing into each other's eyes, deepens the spiritual connection, enhances and prolongs the experience. All the while elevating the spirit of both individuals and the spirit of the couple. This elevated spiritual energy resonates throughout the relationship bringing greater harmony. *This loving resonance is expansive and the loving spirit and energy of the couple touches all that they encounter. Like an enveloping aural embrace.*

> Spiritual Emotional Xperience

Summation

As I stated in the introduction, I developed this technique by combining Tongue Placement with the Cleansing Breath, Taoist and Yogic practices. First let me give a brief description of Tongue Placement. There are three critical points at the roof of the mouth. The first one being at the back and top of the front teeth; this is called the Wind Point. The second is at the very center of the roof of the mouth; this is called the Fire Point. The third is at the back and just in front of the uvula and is called the Water Point. These names make a lot of sense when you are aware of how they correlate to the formation of the body and functioning of the various organs. As Dr. Llaila O. Afrika taught when I took his Certified Holistic Health Consultant course, you can examine any part of the body by dividing it into three segments. These segments correlate to the way the organs and glands are divided Upper, Middle, and Lower. When we consider that the lungs and respiratory system is in the upper portion we get the Wind Point being at the front of the roof of the mouth. And the digestive organs, which in Asian medicine and Tai Chi is called the furnace, is in the middle of the body so that area is the Fire Point. Finally, the reproductive and excretory organs in the pelvic region are represented as the Water Point in the rear of the roof of the mouth. Placing the tongue at either of these points brings energy to the organs at these various parts of the body. Very much like reflexology. *As you read on keep the tongue to the roof of the mouth.*

When studying with Dr. Wayne Chandler he informed us that the most powerful of these points is the Water Point. When you hold your tongue to this point for a bit, your mouth will begin to water and this water will have sweetness to it. He described how when one of his fellow students asked their instructor how often he placed his tongue at this point he responded, "Whenever I'm not talking, eating, drinking or sleeping." When asked what were the effects of doing this Dr. Chandler stated that it basically tunes you in. I pondered this statement for many months while practicing this technique intermittently. Then that magical moment of clarity arrived one day. As I was practicing some breathing techniques I included the Tongue Placement technique, and realized that it changed the depth of the breath significantly. I continued and began examining the full extent of its impact on the breathing apparatus.

This is what I discovered: When you curl your tongue to reach to the rear of the roof of the mouth it pulls and lifts the top and full length of the front of the trachea (windpipe). This expands the dimensions of the trachea dramatically, giving room for a greater volume of air. This greater volume of air goes directly into the lower portion of the lungs pressing down on the diaphragm gently but with vigor. As I explain in the chapter on Fight or Flight vs. Relaxation & Meditation, breathing into the lower portion of the lungs facilitates relaxation and meditation. That magical state of being, where, we are tuned in to all the energies around us. This was indeed a magnificent discovery. Especially when considering how difficult it is for many to learn to change their breathing pattern to one of slower and deeper breathing. All Yoga instructors can attest to that. Knowing how significant this difference is, and how vital the breath is, I had to move immediately to passing on this great gift.

I explained Tongue Placement first because it deals with the first part of the breath, inhalation. But I first learned the Cleansing Breath from Master Yersir Ra Hotep, my first Kemetic Yoga instructor. The Cleansing Breath is relatively simple in that you focus mainly on the exhalation. While lying on the floor in the Mummy Pose, you place your hands on your lower abdomen left hand on top for ladies and right on top for guys. After a full inhalation you slowly and gently exhale making an audible *haah* sound, the way you would if you were trying to steam up a glass or mirror. Making this sound while exhaling actually engages the lower abdominal muscles. This causes the expulsion of a far greater amount of carbon dioxide and stagnant air. Air that for many has sat in the lower recesses of the lungs for years because of shallow upper chest breathing. This too I found very intriguing. So much so I began to think to myself, every breath should be a cleansing breath. Hey, that just makes such perfect sense. After all that's what breathing is all about, getting the good stuff in and the bad stuff out!

This was so profound to me that before I developed the Breath Mastery Technique, and the Breath of Life Clinic I developed and entire exercise series with that at its core. I dubbed it Critical Mass Movement & Breath Mastery. Critical Mass Movement, because many have reached critical mass in their bodies and are in great need of a massive movement, Breath Mastery because of how mastering the breath helps to facilitate that movement. Also poor health and obesity have reached Critical Mass and we are in great need of a Mass Movement toward health. For brevity it is now entitled the Internal Fitness Series™.

> Be diligent and you will gain confidence, stamina and a level of Internal Fitness and health beyond compare.

Chapter 3

Breath of Life Clinic

As part of a good yoga practice there is always a segment of time devoted to breathing exercises. There are various types of breathing exercises that are employed. In this series we are not going to get into the broader array of breathing exercises. We will utilize however not only the Cleansing Breath; as mentioned previously as part of the Breath Mastery Technique, we will also be working with the Breath of Fire. Followed by a short set of Knee Raises. The Knee Raises intensify the toning and strengthening of the abdominal muscles and are a brief introduction to the Internal Fitness Series. Let's get familiar with the Breath of Fire.

Breath of Fire:

During this exercise the mouth will remain closed and both inhalation and exhalation will be done through the nose. Get out the tissue! This is a rapid exercise similar in pace to that of the oral breathing women do during contractions when giving birth. Speaking of Pregnancy none of the exercises in this book should be attempted while pregnant or severely constipated.

- **Place your hands on your abdomen feeling to make sure the breath is focused into the abdomen throughout this exercise.**

- **While seated upright in a chair or in the Lotus Position (Indian style), place the tongue to the back of the roof of the mouth; inhale slowly into nostrils.**

- **Keep the mouth closed; rapidly exhale and inhale through the nostrils as fast as you can as many times as you can for 8-10 seconds into the abdomen.**

- **Relax and breathe normally for a few breaths to regroup.**

- **Repeat rapid exhalation and inhalation for 8-10 seconds; then relax.**

- **Lengthen intervals and practice time as your stamina builds.**

Okay that was fine. That was just a warm up to familiarize you with the Breath of Fire. After you get the hang of it you won't need to place the hands on the abdomen every time. If you need to practice a little more and review the BMT before proceeding to the next section feel free to do so. Now let's get into the Breath of Life Clinic.

Breath of Life Clinic

Alternate between Breath Mastery Technique (BMT), and Breath of Fire (BoF)

- **Complete 3-5 breaths utilizing BMT.**

- **Pause for a 3 count.**

- **Take one full inhalation.**

- **Begin 8-10 seconds BoF.**

- **Fully express the breath, pause for a 3 count.**

- **Complete 3-5 breaths utilizing BMT.**

> The Breath of Life Clinic is designed to replicate the benefits of interval training; using only the breath.

- **Pause for a 3 count.**

- **Take one full inhalation.**

- **Repeat 8-10 seconds BoF.**

- **Fully express the breath, pause for a 3 count.**

- **Repeat 3-5 breaths utilizing BMT.**

- **Pause for a 3 count. Take one full inhalation.**

- **Repeat 8-10 seconds BoF.**

- **Fully express the breath, pause for a 3 count.**

- **Repeat 3-5 breaths utilizing BMT.**

5 Alternating Knee Raises per leg to be performed either seated or standing as slow as possible.

- **Inhale using BMT.**

- **While slowly exhaling with the *haah* sound raise left knee above waste-line with the breath.**

- **Pause for 3 count then lower the leg as you inhale slowly using BMT.**

- **Repeat on the right side.**

- **Repeat left, right sequence for minimum of 5 times per leg.**

- **Relax session concluded.**

Wow, that was exhilarating wasn't it? I trust you had the discipline to complete the entire clinic. If because of a lack of stamina you weren't able to complete the entire sequence this time that's okay as long as you gave it a valiant effort. That's what practice and time are for. And I know you will give it plenty of both. Schedule this clinic for yourself no less than 3 times a day, morning, noon and night. If you are on a serious mission; determined to achieve impressive results in improving your health and well-being, schedule more than that. But don't overdo it; be mindful of your capacity. Please note that the time, intervals and number of breaths outlined are not written in stone. If you have to start with lesser amounts of time and numbers of breaths feel free to do so. This is not about *proving* anything, but it is seriously about *improving* your health and well-being. You have to move at a pace that is comfortable for you and does not strain your body in any way. To help make it easy for you to become acclimated and stay on track be sure to get any of the audio versions of the Internal Fitness Series™. You can listen to it every morning or any time to help you focus and relax while you improve you're breathing and Internal Fitness.

For those who have a higher level of fitness and find the length of the BoF and the number of the BMT to be short and not as challenging as you feel you need for your own progression, feel free to make the necessary adjustments that suit you. The times and number of breaths given are what may be reasonable for someone in the normal health range.

But once again they are not written in stone. You have a better idea of what your body can handle. And please remember that as you practice over time your stamina will increase. So be mindful and increase the numbers and the overall time of the breath clinic as your stamina develops.

> **AS STAMINA BUILDS INCREASE THE NUMBER OF BREATHS AND OVERALL TIME OF THE CLINIC.**

Summation

Studying with Dr. Afrika, was the first time I truly took notice of the term interval training. He informed, that it was the primary if not only guaranteed way to lose weight with exercise. I later learned that elite athletes have been using interval training to boost metabolism, build muscle, increase stamina and shed unwanted pounds.

The way this works is; they set a time period of half an hour or more that starts with a warm up. Then they do 1–2 minutes of high intensity exercise followed by 2–4 minutes of low intensity moderate paced exercise. They will continue alternating these short intervals for the duration of the time set. Ending with the moderate pace as a cool down. The benefits of interval training that have been reported are very powerful. There is a natural increase in the level of human growth hormone. Also, greater muscle development, a drastic increase in metabolism, massive burning of calories and shedding of weight. This is very significant when compared to a regular workout that is steadily paced for the same overall time. By comparison you don't get the increase in human growth hormone or the other dramatic increases mentioned. And there is a far less risk of injury with interval training.

The Breath of Life Clinic is designed to replicate the benefits of interval training, utilizing the breath. The Breath of Life Clinic can be done practically anywhere and anytime without any equipment. This is a transformational, no impact series. From the first time, and every time thereafter you will feel the power of this exercise, and it's ability to give you great inner strength. Since there is no impact there is practically no risk of injury. At worst you will experience a burning in the abdominal muscles you haven't felt in years, if ever.

The Breath of Fire was chosen for this series because it is probably the highest intensity breathing exercise. The reason it is called the Breath of Fire is because it heats up the abdomen rapidly and like nothing else can. That heat then radiates throughout the body. As I mentioned before the abdomen is known in the Eastern culture as the furnace. Where the fire of the body resides and cooks whatever we eat. By intensifying this heat and increasing the amount of oxygen supplied to stoke this fire our digestive and reproductive organs are given a great amount of energy that revitalizes and rejuvenates.

When doing the various practices of Chi Gong, the breath is deep and rhythmic. The movements are fluid, graceful and slow. With the increased amount of oxygen and the lack of vigorous movement, instead of fueling muscle the oxygen fuels the organs. This gentle movement opens the joints and allows for free passage of energy. Waste flows through to the invigorated organs to be removed from the body. This awareness, plus the toning of the abdominal muscles, joined with the benefits of the interval training is the reason for the creation of the Breath of Life Clinic. Be diligent and you will gain confidence, stamina and a level of Internal Fitness and health beyond compare.

Chapter 4

Fight or Flight

vs

Relaxation & Meditation

Now let us examine the lungs. In order to truly overstand the way breath impacts our physiology and our metaphysical being we must study the workings of the lungs. We've often heard the term fight or flight and in human development the Fight or Flight mechanism. This is a tremendous resource for survival. We must have an immediate response to dangerous situations because time is of the essence. But what about the rest of the time, let's explore this.

Fight or flight:

In military training and in many sports depending on the methodology they teach: suck in that gut and stick out that chest. This is the epitome of upper lung breathing. Since we see soldiers and athletes as strong people we imitate this pattern throughout society. We must be aware that the primary purpose of a soldier is to fight or run for cover. In the heat of battle there is or no time for relaxation. When you take a look at how the lungs work in a stressful situation the breathing becomes short and rapid. This rapidly increases the flow of oxygen for a short burst of energy to fuel the muscles for fighting to protect ones self, or fleeing to escape potential harm. This is vital to our very existence. However the fact must be emphasized that this is meant for short-term explosive action. In this process the lungs don't have time to fill up from bottom to top. So this is only an upper respiratory function. Therefore the upper portion of the lungs is known as the fight or flight region.

In addition there is a rush of adrenaline to truly give us explosive capability, and added strength. Obviously this is a highly stressful state within the body. This is a necessary short-term action, not to be continued for extended periods of time. If this state is maintained for extended periods of time it causes the body to deteriorate. We know this is true because we know that fight or flight is an extremely heightened stress level. We also know that stress exacerbates all forms of dis-ease, and severely compromises the immune system. Stress constricts the blood vessels contributing to high blood pressure. In cases where the vessels are already restricted from plaque or cholesterol build up or inflamed this can be disastrous. We wind up with conditions were vessels burst and nerves are inflamed. As we examine the fight or flight scenario shallow breathing stands out as a critical issue that needs addressing.

> **If the highly stressful Fight of Flight state is maintained for extended periods of time it causes the body to deteriorate.**

Shallow Breathing:

The critical issue involving the stress levels that many of us find ourselves in is that shallow breathing is a silent, or in some cases not so silent, epidemic. I would venture to say, the breathing pattern amongst the vast majority is shallow. And as explained in the previous paragraph it maintains heightened stress levels in the body. Many of us live ours lives in a constant state of emergency. There are many negative effects of shallow breathing as a long term breathing pattern. When we live extended periods of our lives with shallow breathing we basically are not getting enough oxygen. Carbon dioxide levels are almost always high. Further we're not getting full use of the entire breathing apparatus. All of which are critical in order to function optimally and stave off dis-ease. Oxygen is so vital and important that one of the first things they do when loading a person on an ambulance is give them oxygen. I remember in the past the first piece of advice given someone when they got angry was to take a deep breath. This works because it diffuses the stressful fight or flight mechanism that is accompanied by shallow breathing. While I'm on the subject of anger management I might as well mention the other piece of advice given which is hold your tongue. When doing Breath Mastery workshops I always mention the fact that the

Breath Mastery Technique is the perfect way to calm anger. It facilitates deep breathing and teaches you how to hold your tongue.

Another aspect of shallow breathing that is not associated with fight or flight is that it is a condition of a sedentary lifestyle. Know any couch potatoes? It's also a common attribute of obesity. In the segment on Internal Massage we will explore how changing the shallow breathing pattern will impact the whole weight debate. Sleep Apnea a deadly condition where a person actually stops breathing for short periods of time is another attribute of obesity. What is not noted is the fact that shallow breathing plays a part in the development of both conditions.

Relaxation & Meditation:

I find it very odd that until I became immersed in the practice of Kemetic Yoga I had not been given a term to describe the lower portion of the lungs. The statement I heard was that this was the relaxation portion. This was a phrase that was new to me and I still haven't heard it used outside of the practice of yoga. Upon further analysis I realized that not only does this region facilitate relaxation, it is vital in facilitating meditation. I don't know if this has been introduced as a term before now, but I want to officially acknowledge this portion as the Relaxation & Meditation portion of the lungs. Whether this is the first time you've heard this or not I beseech each and every one of you to use this term prolifically. This is something that needs to come into the forefront of our consciousness. Like a Mantra the words themselves facilitate their meaning, *relaxation and meditation.* Just using the term will increase its awareness. Making note of this will imprint it into the general knowledge base and get us back to a more natural form of breathing. It will also carry us to greater levels of personnel development.

THE BREATH MASTERY TECHNIQUE IS THE PERFECT WAY TO CALM ANGER.

In today's fast paced two or more jobs needed to make it world, stress is a major factor and way of life. For many of us there seems to be little to no time for relaxation on a regular basis. This is a dire situation as regular relaxation is therapeutic and essential for good health. We can talk about the many conditions that are made worse by a lack of relaxation. Anxiety disorder, panic attacks, hypertension, insomnia, and many others including the many types of cancer. These many conditions are part of a degenerative process. Overtime without adequate time allotted for the body to rest and relax it begins to wear out and break down. Sleep and other forms of relaxation are when the body is in the regenerative stage. Breath work is an enhanced regenerative process. As taught in Chi Gong, when you increase oxygen intake while minimizing movement a far greater amount of oxygen feeds the blood and the internal organs. Making the tissue more supple, invigorating and revitalizing them. Thus enabling them to better remove waste, toxins and bad cells from the body through elimination. Enriching the blood in this manner constantly helps the body to begin anew.

Meditation is relaxation with assertive if not aggressive intent. It helps us transcend stress on a deeper level. Not only do we transcend stress and many emotional and physical conditions, we also achieve spiritual growth. Hence the term made popular in the 1960's Transcendental Meditation. We transcend the constant rightness and chatter of the conscious mind and allow the subconscious to open and develop. Over time and with guided practice the imprinting of the subconscious actually guides the conscious mind. *This is the ultimate version of the psychological term passive aggressive.* The subconscious is where peace and serenity reside; visitations to this place within helps counterbalance all the stressors that diminish immune and regenerative function. Counterbalancing these stressors relieves the body of their impact, and allows it to recuperate and thrive. This is what really goes on when we say boosting the immune system.

I must at this time point out the impact of breath work on two conditions specifically. These two conditions are major health issues of the day. They are High Blood Pressure and Obesity; these two often go hand in hand. Both of these conditions have been scientifically proven to improve with breath work. I am of the opinion that breath work is essential to dealing with these issues. Therefore it is imperative that it be included in any type of protocol for these issues. I mentioned before that Sleep Apnea is a condition common in obese individuals. This condition comes about when there is too much soft tissue in the throat. That could be fatty tissue and or muscles that are not adequately toned. The Breath Mastery Technique and Breath of Life Clinic (BoLC) when practiced regularly can help open the airway and tone the muscles in the throat to help improve the mechanical aspects of this condition. *Is your tongue still in place?*

> # Like a mantra the words themselves
> ## facilitate their meaning.
> # RELAXATION & MEDITATION

Chapter 5

Internal Massage

When we examine the functioning of the breathing process and the various body parts that are actively engaged we see that there is a synchronicity that creates a dynamic series of events. We've already talked about the fight or flight, and relaxation and meditation aspects of the upper and lower portions of the lungs. Now lets examine the lungs and the diaphragm a little further. After that we will explore how the abdominal muscles come into play in the fully engaged breathing process. As we do this we will discuss the impact of these actions on the organs of the digestive system.

The Lungs and Diaphragm:

When looking at the lungs we see that they function much like a bellows. Air enters the top through a tube as the rib cage expands outward. As the lungs fill similar to the bag part of the bellows the lower portion is pulled downward. The muscle that runs horizontally along the bottom of the lungs is called the diaphragm. As the diaphragm aids in the intake of oxygen, (inhalation), in a downward pull it simultaneously presses down on the digestive and reproductive organs beneath it. In a normal breath this press is gentle. As the muscles that pull the rib cage outward and the diaphragm relax the downward press on the organs below the diaphragm is relaxed also. *When we engage the breath fully as with the Breath Mastery Technique the lungs expand more and the downward press on the organs beneath the diaphragm is more substantial.*

When exhaling with the **haah** sound as in the Breath Mastery Technique and the Cleansing Breath the diaphragm actually creates a gentle vacuum action that pulls the lower organs upward. As you can see this facilitates a gentle but very deliberate and dynamic up and down push and pull. Since these organs are filled with liquids and food particles in various stages of digestion, this movement helps with the continuous flow in a timely manner. Doing this on a regular basis keeps down stagnation and accumulation of toxins in these organs. I haven't mentioned the effect this has on the reproductive organs. For women in particular this increase in the flow of oxygen rich blood helps normalize hormone levels. Many women have an excessive menstrual flow due to low oxygen levels in the womb. Increasing oxygen to this area can correct this problem. This in turn boosts health indicators throughout the body especially Iron level and Anemia. For men this increased flow of oxygen rich blood can prevent and alleviate Erectile Dysfunction.

> The downward press on the organs is more substantial and keeps down stagnation and toxin accumulation.

The Abdominal Muscles:

When expressing the breath with the ***haah*** sound we simultaneously engage the muscles of the lower abdomen. When the lower abdominal muscles are engaged they press the organs toward the back and lift the belly. Utilizing the Breath Mastery Technique puts the lower abdominal muscles to work. Without regular use and exercise the abdominal muscles become like rubber bands that have lost their elasticity. When we look at the abdominals we see that they are a band of muscles that run vertically from the sternum to the pubis. Like all muscles they must be exercised regularly to stay tone. In a sedentary lifestyle the muscles lack tone and eventually become distended. This allows for the development of what we call a gut. I just mentioned the upward and downward motion of the diaphragm; well the abdominals facilitate a front to back push. The combination of the two actions creates a gentle but vigorous massaging of all the organs that sit between the diaphragm and the pelvic floor. This is why to the surprise of many; deep breathing exercises aid digestion and helps with elimination, alleviating constipation. *When you fully empty the accumulated waste the weight of the waste goes too and subsequently the body drops pounds. In principle this is why deep breathing exercises in general, the Breath Mastery Technique and the Breath of Life Clinic in particular, causes weight loss and normalizes body mass.*

Let's give this a little more in depth but simple analysis:

In using the BMT you create a gentle, but vigorous and extensive massage. This massaging process effectively squeezes out various fluids and matter that these organs have processed for elimination. Facilitating efficient moving to and through the intestines for a more productive, less sluggish (constipation) bowel movement. The blood is invigorated with oxygen, which in turn oxygenates the organs fully. This oxygen enlivens the organs stimulating them to do their jobs more efficiently and effectively. In this process the tissues of the organs are made suppler. They are massaged and manipulated to encourage the flow of fluids and matter through them. Squeezing gently makes them more pliable and gives them a youthful texture. When organs don't move they become stiff. Much like the rest of the body. With the constant buildup of toxins and being stretched beyond their natural capacity the skin (tissue) that makes up these organs hardens. Even worse is when there is such a buildup that either the toxins or the mutated cells they assist in creating, called cancer, begin to eat away at this tissue.

This process revitalizes, reenergizes and renews the organs. Over time shallow breathing, paying little attention to the abdominal muscles, the lower abdominals in particular, allows them to become distended. Much like a rubber band that is fully stretched and has lost its elasticity. Unlike a rubber band however the muscles can regain elasticity. Muscles have memory and know their purpose. With many people these muscles have gotten so stretched and distended that the belly has become huge and bloated. Without this massage, bloating and an expansive amount of space is allowed, wherein waste accumulates continuously. *The digestive organs are basically a series of bags along a long digestive tube. They each hold and process various constituents that pass through them. However the abdominal cavity is allowed to expand to great proportions in many people today. Instead of small or normal size bags that fill and empty regularly, they become large bags filled with toxins and waste that continue to accumulate.* Accumulating to the point that they are not able to function adequately. They become clogged with gunk, and toxins that cause cells to mutate. With the inadequacy of oxygen free radicals proliferate. Cells missing an oxygen molecule, they basically steal oxygen molecules from other cells in sheer desperation for their own survival. So the body is beset upon itself, because of inadequacy in this whole process.

Our bodies as landfills:

> Lose the waste
> Lose the weight

Constant overeating and perpetual accumulation of waste and toxic buildup, is very much the like landfill process. The body becomes like a landfill with the accumulation of all kinds of debris and poisons. Parasitic organisms are like the scavengers that are always present at a landfill.

Hovering, flying, crawling, scratching, digging and looking for some type of debris or decaying substance to thrive on. Parasites, bacteria and cancers are scavengers in the body that consume the host while seeking waste to thrive on. Waste that shouldn't even be present in the body. If the waste isn't present the risk of these parasitic organisms, worms and such is minimal. Which is also why we need various components in our **LIVE~IT**, not **diet**, that create a wholesome clean environment that makes it inhospitable for parasites and so on. We will learn more about these in the Biodynamic Nutrition book.

Back to the abdominal muscles, this breathing process will change the breathing pattern; the abdominal muscles will become more tone over time. Aiding in the digestive process by squeezing out these toxins. As important: once these abdominal muscles become taught, and no longer distended, there will be less space for the accumulation of waste. Squeezing out toxins and eliminating waste creates an exponential effect on removal of toxins and toning of the abdominal muscles. Reviving the effective and efficient waste removal system you were born with.

I find a certain popular television show about weight loss competition disturbing. I was always surprised at the disappointment of the contestants. After the second or third week they reach a point where it was difficult to lose weight at the same rate as the first couple of weeks. My analysis of this is that it takes time for the type of exercises being utilized to get the metabolism going. Also these exercises don't massage the organs milking waste from them. Even more so, the initial part of their weight loss was part of a process that I call *the cessation of perpetual waste buildup*. As time goes on and we overeat constantly there is a continuous gradual waste accumulation. When the rate of intake is greater than the rate of elimination there is buildup. If this is a constant then the waste accumulation is perpetual. Changing the eating habits; i.e. lowering the amount of intake slows down or stops the perpetual accumulation and we begin "loosing weight." After a couple of weeks this levels out. The metabolic rate has not risen substantially enough in this brief time frame. The organs are not being squeezed to continuously move the massive accumulation in the bodies of these people. They stop loosing and in some case begin gaining again. The weight loss becomes stalled.

If they were to employ a perpetual waste loss system as described in this series I would venture to say that the weight loss would not stall but be continual and not stagnate. Further these people would achieve a higher quality of health in a shorter period of time, because their bodies would be less put upon by waste. Their stamina would increase dynamically with the increased oxygen intake, and the organs will be more invigorated. This greater amount of oxygen will be utilized to nourish the blood and organs instead of being used to fuel muscle for excessive and exhausting movement. The types of exercises used on the show are specifically designed to make people sweat and burn off calories. Burning off calories is a good idea, however squeezing out toxins and getting rid of waste is a more functional way of getting rid of pounds. *Because, once you get rid of the waste there goes the weight. After all, the weight is the weight of the accumulated waste in the organs and pockets of fat. Like bags of garbage that have yet to be carried out; emptying these organs of accumulated waste and depleting the pockets of fat is a more practical strategy.*

Focused moving of accumulated waste form the body, through the eliminative process, will cause this weight loss process to be more efficient and effective. Further, invigorating the organs that process waste, both new and accumulated will dramatically increase the metabolic rate. Especially in the case of people trying to lose a lot of weight. As long as they are diligent in maintaining the nutritional aspect by following the Circadian Rhythm, as explained in the Biodynamic Nutrition book. Along with the Breath Mastery Technique, Breath of Life Clinic, and the exercises in the Internal Fitness Book. These exercises facilitate the squeezing of the organs and toning of the abdominal muscles to help the body maintain itself optimally. This is the mastery of the basics of life, and your body, in order to achieve the mastery of life itself.

The abdominal muscles will become more tone over time, and will aid in the digestive process by squeezing out toxins and waste.

Parasites, bacteria and cancers are scavengers in the body that consume the host while seeking waste to thrive on.

Final Thoughts

I've heard that the optimal number of breaths per minute is 8. Well in the traditions of the ancient Egyptians, those who were considered masters of the life process functioned on 2 slow, deep, long breaths per minute. They were said to be in a constant state of a walking trance. When achieving this state humans are said to be functioning in the more God like state of man. As compared to the more animal like nature of man with constant shallow more rapid breathing. Just as the fight or flight breathing stresses and causes the body to rapidly deteriorate. Slower deeper breathing maintains the integrity and youthfulness of the body.

It is vitally important that the Breath Mastery Technique and the Breath of Life Clinic become an integral part of your life's routine. Set a schedule for yourself in the beginning and stick to it. Document the times and amount of time practiced. Making sure to note the various changes and nuances you experience in your body. Share these experiences with family and friends, as it will be beneficial to all in your group dynamic. Create dialog and practice sessions with family members. Do the same with your various social groups, coworkers, church, organization members and so on. Maintain your regular schedule, and use the Breath Mastery Technique and Tongue Placement throughout the day as well. Be fully aware that this is a valuable and vital tool for human development and treat is as such. The same goes for the other books in this series.

Teach these techniques to your children and grandchildren. We must teach the youth and give them tools that will ensure them a healthy and fulfilled life as unfettered and unencumbered as possible. Share this knowledge with your coworkers and organization members. When you give this book as a gift to someone who you know may be struggling and needs a breath of fresh air, you may even save his or her life.

My blog is internalfitnesstrainer.wordpress.com. Please follow me on the web. I would love to hear your stories of how this book and my work in general help you and those around you. If I am in your area speaking or presenting please come and see me live and in person. It is my deepest hope that like my parents I have helped all those that are in need of my unique ability to do so.

Breathe deeply, love intensely and live well.

BOOK

TWO

BIODYNAMIC

NUTRITION

Biodynamic Nutrition

Table of Contents

Introduction

Book Two of the Trinity

Oxygen   Nutrition   Exercise

Fuels and **O**xygenates **O**ptimally **D**aily, this is the meaning of the word food. If what you are putting into your mouth and body does not fit this criteria it is not **FOOD**, it is Stuff. Stuff is devoid of many of foods original components and lacks life, therefore cannot sustain life. Stuff is toxic and either inappropriate or unfit for human consumption. Some Stuff like cow's milk is designed for consumption by other animals therefore inappropriate for human consumption. Many processed so-called foods are not only unfit but down right hazardous and even poisonous. Stuff lives up to its name; it stuffs the body with waste misshaping it, expanding it to enormous proportions. Stuff accumulates, coagulates, congests, and destroys the body system-by-system, organ-by-organ, and gland-by-gland. From now on examine everything you put into your mouth and on peoples plates. Are you eating **FOOD** or are you eating **Stuff**?

Food must be whole, fresh, energetic, life engaging and enhancing. The body has to reconstitute things that have been altered in order to process them. Therefore elements removed in the refining process are pulled from other parts of the body, depleting them throughout the body. Refined carbohydrates turn into sugar, which ferments into alcohol, a solvent creating further problems throughout the body. Know the benefits of and the purpose of everything you put into your body. Gather knowledge so you can make conscious decisions with an awareness of the potential outcome. Use this awareness to guide your decisions toward a positive outcome instead of an undesirable condition.

The intent of this book in this three book series is to begin that education. First you will learn the Circadian Rhythm. This is a very basic Biorhythm that is not widely taught. Which is very unfortunate as it lets you know when to eat what type of food. Following that you will learn about food combining. As you view and review the Food Combining Chart it will make a lot of sense as it flows with the logic of the Circadian Rhythm. Next, the importance of water to a biodynamic **LIVE~IT**, followed by the extremely vital process of chewing and it's impact on digestion. As we build on your knowledge in a logical progression, the Vital Properties of highly nutritious foods will be discussed. You will then be given a list of vibrant foods, many of which you are already familiar with. In the Foods & Frequency chapter you will gain clarity from the explanation of how increasing the quantity of these high quality foods will create abundant health. Make sure to use the foods in this chapter to create your grocery list. A good idea would be to do this immediately as you read through the first time. There will be little talk about what not to eat and a lot about what foods to eat and how often. To support your basic food intake the chapters on Smoothies, Juicing, Sprouts, Soups, and The Art of Snacking™, will provide ways to continuously increase the immune boosting, healing aspects of your **LIVE~IT**.

Here are a few tips to consider while reading this book. Your body is a perpetual motion machine; keep it moving. To keep moving vibrantly you must maintain consistent fueling of this machine; you never want to run out of gas. Therefore, smaller meals every 2-3 hours is better than three larger heavy meals per day. This keeps the metabolism running smoothly. And, avoids the crash that happens when the body is stuffed and has to redirect much of the blood flow to the digestive tract to deal with sudden overload.

If you want to skip right into Foods and Frequency or one of the latter chapters to speed you on your way feel free to do so. However make sure to immediately return to the beginning and read through to the end. The information is presented in a logical progression that supports a fundamental grasp on the subject that will give you confident, practical expertise. This information is invaluable; you and your family or group will find yourselves referring back to it constantly for years to come.

> **We now have to be reeducated on how to live a healthy and natural life.**

Chapter 1

Circadian Rhythm

We must grasp the basic fact that we eat to fuel our bodies. We may think otherwise or have had our perspectives warped by societal, emotional and peer pressures. However the body doesn't move away from this mere fact of functionality. It is impossible to deny that we eat impulsively and without conscious intent for the most part today. This leaves us open to the onslaught of the many maladies that accompany over consumption. Especially since we stuff ourselves with things that our bodies do not recognize as food. Processed, synthesized, wrapped in plastic and full of preservatives, Stuff that has little or no nutritional value. While the number one drug on the planet, *sugar*, may make these things taste good it adds to the collection of poisonous content. Making good food choices is one of the critical pieces of the puzzle. We must also be aware of not only what to eat but also, when to eat, and what to eat when. Our bodies have various rhythms and cycles that it follows in order to maintain optimal health.

When life began for us in the rain forests of Africa we were attached to the land and our environment. It wasn't difficult for us to flow with the rhythms and cycles of our bodies. They were and still are intrinsically connected to that environment and it's rhythms and cycles. When we got up in the morning with the sunrise we would reach up into the trees and pick fruit that glistened with the dew drops of a bright new day. We would take walks and stretch. And we would squat two or three times and relieve ourselves. Automatically upon rising gravity was in full affect. The foods from the latter part of the previous day had been processed its waste was ready to be returned to the soil. The fruit not lonely quenches our thirst but also give us quick energy to start the day. As the day would wear on our eyes would shift from looking up at the morning sun and the glistening jewels of the fruit trees. Shifting to eye and trunk level leaves, stalks, grains and the various seed pods, legumes, nuts and so on. They would give us sustained energy that would keep us satiated so we could continue our chores throughout midday and early after noon. Before twilight our eyes would follow the setting sun and we would look toward the horizon and about the ground for more leaves and pumpkins, squash, and root vegetables. These would be our soups for supper and dinner that would end our day as we prepare to follow the sun to bed for a restful rejuvenating sleep. Being so removed from nature and being so well educated about practically every subject, except the most vital, *how to live a healthy and natural life.* We now have to be reeducated on this most delicate and previously simple way of life. I won't go on an environmentalist tirade, but I will mention that living with a true connectedness to nature is not only beneficial to our bodies but the planet as well. Indigenous cultures that modern man, with his industrialized mind, sees as backwards have survived for hundreds of thousands of years. Knowing that we are to be stewards of the land. And further it is the greatest value that our children will inherit, lest we undermine and destroy their inheritance.

The *Circadian Rhythm is the rhythmic cycle that deals with what types of food should be eaten at what interval of the day.* It also deals with when we should not be eating certain foods and not eating at all. *No cookies or candy in bed.* The Circadian Rhythm is all about the flow of food into and out of the body. Managing food intake with this very basic biorhythm will allow one to master process of elimination (pun intended). All the while, moving one further along the process of mastering the life experience. Without adhering to this it becomes very difficult to manage health and the aging process in a reasonable fashion. Constipation is the process in which waste matter gets clogged in the body by various means. The toxins that are to be eliminated on a regular and timely basis begin to accumulate and cause the body to go into various states of dis-ease. The area of the body wherein this accumulation starts and is more pronounced is the waste line; fashionably referred to as the waistline, notice the change in spelling. Even the language betrays our awareness. There has long been a saying, " disease begins in the colon." The previous sentences tell why this saying is very true. This is how diverticulitis, hypertension, cancers, autoimmune, circulatory and vascular diseases and obesity to name a few of the modern plagues begin.

I've tried to give you a perspective from our basic natural adaptation and explain some of what happens when we ignore how we are designed. As I said earlier in the Breath Mastery book, in order to master a thing, you first have to master the most basic aspects of that thing. In order to master life you must first master the basic principles upon which it is built. The Circadian Rhythm is a major fundamental principle of life **period.** Here is how it works. The 24-hour day is broken up into three 8-hour intervals. From 4 am to 12 pm the body is in the eliminative phase. From 12 pm to 8 pm it's in the ingestion phase. From 8 pm to 4 am it's in the absorption phase.

Circadian Rhythm Phases

> **4 am – 12 pm Elimination Phase**
> **12 pm – 8 pm Ingestion Phase**
> **8 pm – 4 am Assimilation Phase**

4 am – 12 pm   **Elimination Phase**

Upon rising the body is in the Elimination Phase. There are certain measures that are important to facilitating proper and adequate elimination. There are also measures necessary to quickly replenish the body during this phase without interrupting this vital biorhythm. To alkalize and hydrate the body upon rising one should drink water that is room at temperature with the juice of half a lemon or lime, if lemon is not available. Lemon Water as compared to commercial alkaline water is more alive. It not only alkalizes it provides vitamins, minerals, the two main electrolytes the body needs, sodium and potassium, antioxidants, and bio-flavinoids. Additionally when the lemon is squeezed it ruptures cells in the skin that sprays oils and flavinoids into the air. This freshens the air and invigorates the respiratory system. Talk about starting your day with a blast.

> **The Circadian Rhythm**
> **is a fundamental**
> **principle of life.**

Only fruits and berries or the same combined with greens in Smoothies should be eaten this early in the day. This provides additional water, lots of enzymes and digests within 30 minutes. Simple sugars provide quick energy; bulk and fiber, to move previously digested matter through the intestines and colon. Fruits and berries carry the seeds of life for the next generation of plants. This natural casing for the seeds has enough water content to germinate the seeds and start them on their way to sprouting and growing into small plants. Another part of the adaptive process that makes sure there is adequate dispersal of varying plant life is that the fruit is enticing to animals. Animals (like us) eat the fruit including the seed. As they move about the fruit encourages quick elimination. The seeds don't get digested and are dropped with a compliment of fecal compost to fertilize the growth of the new seedlings once they emerge from the soil.

Along with the enzymes and water content fruits and berries contain soluble fiber. Soluble fiber maintains water and lubricates the intestines and colon for smooth movement of waste the following morning. The bulk takes up space and pushes out the digested waste the day the fruit is eaten. The morning is the principle time for elimination in a normal functioning human body. Modern lifestyle, demands people get up on the run, causing many to skip taking time for elimination. This causes chronic constipation, obesity and precipitating dis-ease especially after teenage years when metabolism naturally slows down. Unfortunately, for those who are either trained or allowed to become addicted to overeating and eating processed Stuff, at a young age, this starts even earlier. One of the reasons we see Type II Diabetes in children today.

> **Lemon Water compared to commercial alkaline water is more vital and alive.**

Not eating breakfast or eating things other than fresh fruit causes chronic constipation, obesity and precipitating dis-ease. Things such as processed cereal grains: donuts, waffles or pancakes with syrup, grits, eggs, bacon, and sausage that are typical in today's **diet**. Instead of eating heavy foods such as these for breakfast, have three or more pieces of fruit. If you must, have one or two of the heavier foods for brunch between 10 am and 12 pm. Work consciously toward eventually eating just fruits and drinking Smoothies in the morning. This must be done in a manner that is comfortable for you. If you have to make the transition slowly, do so. Start with a few days per week. This may be a drastic lifestyle change for many. So acclimate yourself carefully to avoid the yo-yo struggle of dieting. *This is not a weight loss plan, but living life as it was naturally intended for optimal health.* You should experience a minimum of two or three full bowel movements daily. And these should take place primarily between the hours of 4 am and 12 pm.

> **This is not a weight loss plan; this is living life as nature intended for optimal health.**

12 pm – 8 pm   Ingestion Phase

In this phase of the digestive process, the heavier, slower digested, more protein and higher insoluble fiber foods are eaten. These foods are more complex and need more time to digest because of their density, and insoluble fiber has less water than soluble fiber. This denser fiber requires that we actually increase our water intake. Which is why an hour or more after a meal we are thirsty. Though the requirement for water is greater that does not mean we should drink water with our meal. If we chew our food as outlined in the chapter on Chewing and Saliva we won't feel the need to drink while eating. Remember drinking water while eating dilutes the digestive juices and may lead to constipation. After food has moved through the stomach into the small intestines drinking water will not slow the process as it does prior to it leaving the stomach. This is also why our ancestors in their infinite wisdom began a custom that we should continue. *Making soups* from these foods adds water to them during preparation, which helps them to begin breaking down and quenches our thirst while eating without diluting the digestive juices.

The types of foods eaten during this time period are the parts of the plant other than the fruit. Nuts and seeds for their protein, oils and fiber; legumes, (beans and peas), for their protein, fiber, vitamins and minerals. Roots and tubers are eaten for their minerals, starch and fiber; grains for their starch, fiber, vitamins and minerals. Plants store nutrients in these parts in order to survive dormant periods so there is little need for much water content. Since these foods have less water content they store for longer periods of time without being refrigerated. Unlike fruits and berries with their greater amount of enzymes and water. And by comparison they take longer to break down in the body. Which is why they shouldn't be combined with fruits and berries. This could cause a conflict in the digestive tract that can lead to gas, poor absorption, and a number of health issues.

A few exceptions to this rule are; Papayas, Avocado, and leaves. Papaya has the most powerful plant enzyme, **papain**, which can break down even meat in the digestive tract. Avocado because of its oils, and leaves because they have fiber and high chlorophyll content can be consumed with many other types of food, without causing a conflict. Because of the fact that insoluble fiber doesn't get digested these foods don't need the volume of enzymes that fruits and berries have. Its cellulose fiber serves as the internal broom for the intestines and colon. Unlike their seed carrying counterparts these foods pull more water from the body. Cellulose fiber needs to be kept hydrated as it moves through the digestive tract less it get stuck. This is the reason we drink water later, after our food has left the stomach. These foods impart their nutrients gathered for the long-term growth and health of the plant for our bodies to store in the liver for lasting energy and new cellular growth.

8 pm – 4 am   Assimilation Phase

The Assimilation Phase is key in determining how well we followed our bodies' needs during the Elimination and Ingestion Phase. We must eat our fruits and drink our Smoothies in the morning, and have good eliminations. Eat enough nutrient packed **FOOD** throughout the day and drink enough water. Then we will be able to get a good nights rest. During the Assimilation Phase our bodies are absorbing the nutrients from the food we ate earlier. Waste and toxins are being swept up, bound and moved forward for evacuation in the morning. New cells are being formed; old cells are being carried out. These are the primary things that should happen while we are asleep. This is why we wake up feeling refreshed and renewed. Because that is exactly what you are by this process, refreshed and renewed.

If you awaken sluggish and tired it's a clear sign that you didn't follow the Circadian Rhythm. If you eat heavy foods late at night you short-circuit the entire process. This causes a restart of the digestive process past the appropriate hour. Energy that should be getting stored for the first part of your new day and long-term growth doesn't get stored. Your body is using energy throughout the night to process food in the stomach, small intestines and other organs. This matter should be moving its way through the large intestines on its way to the colon. Also these organs should be resting. The heart has to pump this digesting matter through the body without the aid of movement and gravity. Both of which are helpful when food is consumed during the active part of the day. All this churning through the night and not storing energy is why many wake up sluggish and tired. Instead of feeling refreshed.

Each stage of the digestive process is the foundation for the next. The better you adhere to the Circadian Rhythm the easier it will be for your body from one stage to the next. You can have smooth sailing from one interval to the next or a downward spiral to discomfort and compromised health. Read on and learn more about the properties of various foods and which items in particular have enhanced benefits. As you grasp this information you will make wiser choices, have less questions and begin living the answers.

> Can you raise healthy cows on human milk?
> Why are we told you can raise healthy humans
> on cow's milk? Cows milk, is for baby cows,
> human milk is for baby humans.

> If you weren't born a cow you shouldn't
> be trying to grow up to be one.

Chapter 2

Food Combining Chart

When looking at the Food Combining Chart, the first we notice is that fruits are at the very beginning. This flows with the Circadian Rhythm. This chart gives clear definitive information on the foods that should not be combined as well as the foods that compliment each other. The reason we don't combine certain foods is because of the differing ways they process in the body. Foods that are on top are the foods that should be eaten primarily from 4-12 am. These foods process quickly in the body. Foods in the lower portion of the chart are the foods that should be eaten during the latter part of the day and process slower. Keeping them separated preventions conflicting reactions in the body and allows for better absorption of nutrients. Notice also that melons are to be eaten alone. Included in this book is a description of the Watermelon Flush. If watermelon is not available actually any melon will do you will just have to eat more of them to accomplish the flush. Half a melon of the smaller variety makes a great breakfast that will consistently aid waste removal and weight loss.

Copy this chart and place it on the front of the refrigerator. If you use cookbooks another good idea would be to place a copy in there. This tool be a clear reminder that will make high quality meal and snack planning effortless. The information on this chart may be unfamiliar as it is not general knowledge. Even when it gets taught it winds up being distorted and not adhered to, because of habits and eating patterns that are ingrained. As you make food choices be mindful of the various combinations and make adjustments accordingly. *No fruit for dessert after a heavy meal.*

As you make these adjustments you will be amazed at how great you will feel. You will feel lighter in your body and spirit and have a clearer mind. You will constantly be encouraged as the compliments will lift your spirit and let you know you are on the right track. Questions and statements like, "You really look great these days, did you lose weight?" "You seem to have a glow about you." No burdensome thoughts of becoming debilitated with age, concerned about who will take care of you. Rejoicing, knowing that **you** will take care of **yourself** and age gracefully. *Free at last, free at last Thank God Almighty, Free At Last.*

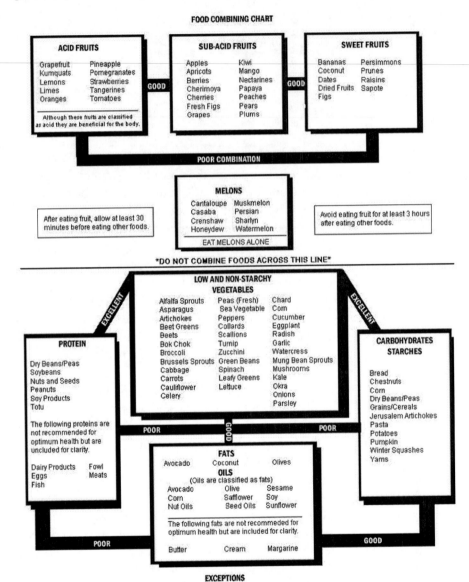

Food combining chart

Chapter 3

Water

Upon rising gravity is in full effect. We all have to go practically before our feet hit the floor. Immediately after releasing so much water first thing, it must be replenished. The best way to do this is by slowly drinking a glass of room temperature water with the juice of half a lemon added. The body processes whatever we ingest at 98.6 degrees or it's present temperature at the time. If you drink cold water it will shock the digestive and nervous systems. This stresses the body unnecessarily, and forces it to work to heat up the water so it can be assimilated. Remember anything that slows down the digestive process can contribute to constipation. *The reason for the lemon is that it alkalizes the body and replenishes the electrolytes, sodium and potassium along with adding other nutrients such as bioflavinoids.* Interesting terms electrolytes and bioflavinoids. I like to say electrolytes light up the body's electricity and bioflavinoids add flavor to life. Make sure that as you take your time drinking to swish thoroughly before swallowing. The digestive reason will be explained shortly. Notice immediately when running your tongue over your teeth the freshness in your mouth. So much for morning breath. This should be done before brushing. There are beneficial cultures in your mouth in the morning that will aid digestion. And that feeling of freshness in your mouth will travel through the digestive tract.

Water is second only to oxygen as far as elements for life. Depending on the age and condition the human body is composed of 80% to 65% water. The 80% is first because we start out fully hydrated at the beginning of life. That's why baby's bottoms and the rest of their bodies are so soft. Water is so crucial an element; we can only live a few days without it. It is

WATER IS SECOND ONLY TO OXYGEN AS FAR AS ELEMENTS FOR LIFE.

essential to all bodily functions and is present in every cell. It hydrates, lubricates and keeps things moving and functioning. Without it life as we know it would not be possible. Just to backtrack a bit on oxygen. Even water would not be possible without oxygen. Its molecular makeup is H_2O. That is 2 parts hydrogen and one part oxygen. That's probably why it is so vital and nearly as vital as oxygen itself as it is composed of oxygen.

The need for adequate intake of water throughout life is a basic principle of life. A major portion of the ailments that we are faced with have a level of dehydration at their core. It should be noted that as we get older the amount of water content in the body decreases. At the same time the number of health related issues that have some type of dehydration aspect to them increase. That's why we say, "*old and dried up.*" Adequate re-hydration can have a positive impact on conditions with dehydration at their core. I would advise anyone to do a search on the Internet on Water Therapy.

We're constantly hearing that we need to drink so many ounces of water per day. This is our primary way of getting water into the body. There are two other factors we need be aware of. The secondary way of getting water into the body, and the fact that processed sugar in all it's stages and forms dries out tissue and dehydrates the body. The secondary means of water consumption is through our foods. Fruits that start our day have an abundance of water content that is combined with fiber and nutrients. The uptake of that water is actually better than when we drink water alone. Raw vegetables such as sprouts, salads, and veggie sticks also provide good amounts of water. The water in these fresh items is more bio available because of their alkalinity. Increasing fresh fruit and vegetable intake, juicing, sprouting, making Smoothies, and soups are ways of increasing water intake and absorption. This manner of increased water intake is more conducive to the digestive process as it practically guarantees the addition of saliva to the ingestion process. With adequate chewing saliva is mixed in so the body recognizes this water as food. And by the way though we separate if from the rest of what we call food; **water is food.** In isolation water is also a solvent. When we drink water alone we should always swish a good amount of it in our mouths before swallowing to add saliva. If you have a problem with swishing, just hold it in your mouth a few seconds. It's not as effective as the swishing but it does activate the salivary glands. The same goes for juices, swishing is like chewing without the grinding part, to begin the digestive process.

> DEPENDING ON AGE AND CONDITION THE HUMAN BODY IS COMPOSED OF 80% TO 65% WATER.

Another good habit is to swish after eating; this rinses food particles from between the teeth. Removing them from the mouth so they don't cause tooth decay and adds saliva so they can be digested. *A natural mouthwash made by either boiling or soaking 20-30 Cloves in 8 ounces of water is perfect for this, it also rids the body of parasites.* Drinking water while eating should be discouraged as this dilutes the digestive juices. Anything that slows the digestive process can cause constipation and with it the accumulation of toxins and waste. As you read earlier it is especially important to drink a glass of room temperature water with the juice of half a lemon upon rising before brushing your teeth. After brushing eat fresh fruit to break your overnight fast. This supplies the body with adequate water and quick energy for this stage of the Circadian Rhythm. Fresh fruit has non-refined simple sugars that provide us quick energy.

> **Without adequate water the blood thickens and moves slower becoming heavier with waste, like a cesspool.**

Another aspect of adequate water intake is it keeps the blood from becoming thick and sticky. Without enough water the blood thickens and moves slower becoming heavier with waste, like a cesspool. This doesn't allow for the free uptake of oxygen. Water is so vital to maintaining all tissue. Inadequate intake and absorption has continuously expanding long-term negative effects. Skin both inside and out becomes dry and leathery, hardening and loosing elasticity. Cartilage and viscous fluids are less spongy and fluid. Space between the bones decreases and nerves become pinched. Bones shrink and become brittle. Tendons and ligaments become tighter and tighter so joints and movement become stiffer. Arteries, veins and nerves become hardened, pressurized, filled with various types of waste and tear or burst. Cells are deprived of oxygen and mutate to form rot within the body.

This brings us to the other major consideration in regards to water in the body: holding on to it. The opposite end that has become so critical that it must be given attention. To stress how important it is to hold onto the water that we are going to great lengths to assimilate and experience the wondrous benefits thereof we must examine the effects of sugar.

!!!SUGAR!!!

Sugar is the number one drug on the planet. And the world's addiction for it has changed the entire course of humanity over the last 600 years. Need I mention the slave trade and sugar plantations? Though some external conditions have changed, on a body-by-body physiological level things have gotten worse. All of the changes in the body mentioned in the previous paragraphs are due in large degree to the consumption of refined sugar. Whether it is in cakes, pies, donuts, and other confections, or so-called soft drinks, which are really hard on the body. Or in it's chemical precursor refined white flour, or it's eventual chemical solvent outcome alcohol. It sucks water and minerals from all the tissues of the body with extreme prejudice, and without discrimination or overlooking a single molecule. You need to think about what you're doing at the start of your day, as it is a microcosmic event that will follow through out your day and life. Coffee with sugar, donuts, Danishes, pancakes with syrup. While you feed this addiction it is feeding on you.

It's time for a wake up call. Some things just have to be said. You will notice in my writing I'm not going into great detail about the various ailments, their causes and cures. When you deal with the basic principles of how the body functions you begin to master the life experience and rise above them all. I would like to focus purely on the positive and give concise powerful information for you to assimilate into your vibrant new life. Information that jump-starts your day, like beginning with the Breath Mastery Technique and that very refreshing glass of Lemon Water. Starting your illuminated new day. This is how I want to help you shift into greater health and Internal Fitness.

> **SOFT DRINKS ARE HARD ON THE BODY AND A MAJOR CAUSE OF DIABETES.**

> When you deal with the basic principles of how the body functions you begin to master the life experience and rise above sickness and affliction.

Chapter 4

Saliva & Chewing

What can I say about spit? Typically the word spit is the first thing that comes to mind and out of a person's mouth when asked; What do they think of when they hear the word saliva? This spontaneous translation does a lot in diminishing the truly significant value of this very dynamic liquid concoction secreted by the salivary glands. Saliva has several very critical functions that when taken for granted can cause minor and major discomfort within the body. Saliva is part of the first stage of the digestive process. The other part of that stage is chewing.

> Blenders, food processors and juicers are mechanical chewers.

We are starting with saliva because even before we start to chew the salivary glands are already at work *making our mouths water*. It is a lubricant that coats the throat and mixes in with food particles to aid their traveling through the esophagus and into the stomach. For that reason it is mostly water and some mucous. It is also composed of the enzyme amylase that begins the break down of carbohydrates for digestion.

Next lets discuss chewing or mastication as it is scientifically called. In the chapter on the Breath Mastery Technique in the Breath Mastery book I explained how my mother used to tell us that instead of chewing all we did was cut and swallow. And how when explaining this to a family when I was a Barber, a pre-teen got tagged with the nickname, "Cut n Swallow." Well other than a chastising by my mother or a joke on someone, chewing your food adequately is a very serious matter. There is a cascading effect that takes place. If you don't chew adequately you have to try to swallow chunks. These chunks of food can get stuck in the throat and cause choking, *Heimlich maneuver anyone*. If there isn't enough saliva to ease its flow what you're attempting to swallow can be drying and abrasive to the esophagus.

Food that reaches the stomach in large chunks takes longer to break down and become taxing on the digestive system. If you eat animal flesh it can lead to more dire circumstance, as the various bacteria that reside inside flesh can be extremely toxic. Poorly digested meat putrefies (rots) in the body, causing the growth of even more dangerous bacteria. Ever see a decaying carcass along the roadway, or afloat in a waterway. In addition to the bacteria dead animal flesh also harbors many harmful parasites. If the animal had parasites you become their new host. Many parasites escape inspection before going on the grocery shelf.

Adequate chewing minimizes these risks. Exposing these contagions to enzymes present in saliva, acid in the stomach, enzymes, antibodies and lymph present in the blood and other parts of the gastro-intestinal tract. Plus taking such a long time to process lends itself to constipation and the repetitive short-circuiting of the Circadian Rhythm. Compounding the problem, a lot of inadequately digested food becomes fat deposits. We also miss out on the added alkalinity of saliva. Without adequate alkalinity the entire system becomes acidic. Acidity is a precursor for many maladies and like stress it exacerbates these issues.

When you have chewed your food enough there will be significant saliva mixed into the bolus. Bolus, that's a strange name for chewed food isn't it. Before you swallow, it should feel like you have a mouth full of soup. Having chewed your food adequately it will be easy to swallow. Have you ever watched some people stretch and crane their neck trying to swallow a chunk of something they haven't fully chewed? Then they grab a glass of water to *wash it down.* **Don't do this.** This can potentially lead to major health problems as they age. I've explained what happens when you don't chew your food adequately, and why you shouldn't drink water while you're eating. Most people who do either of these tend to do both. If both of these are bad habits with bad outcomes when they are combined the issues become seriously compounded. First, in not chewing the food you have not started the break down of the carbohydrates. Then what little saliva that is added is immediately diluted. Followed by the diluting of stomach acid. Another bad habit that many have that practically insures that they will have these two is over stuffing the mouth every time they put food in. If you have to open wide enough for the Dentist to work on your teeth to get the shovel, I mean spoon or fork in, there is simply too much for the mouth to reasonably manage. There isn't enough room for the food to be maneuvered and chewed before your jaws are tired and want to push this stuff down. In all actuality this is disrespectful of the food and your body. Doing these things set's the body up for major digestive issues. Eating should not make you thirsty. Adequately chewed food satiates the body fulfilling the appetite and quenching the thirst.

Since I've mentioned the combination of poor chewing and drinking water, let's talk about a way to break this habit. Instead of focusing on the breaking of a habit I like to focus on a new healthier habit. That way we don't continually give energy to the old habit and keep it alive. This new habit will ignite a healthy passion for food and it's many smells, tastes and textures. The first thing I want you to do at the beginning of your meal is take 5 to 10 breaths using the Breath Mastery Technique. After you're relaxed smell the food, you might want to close your eyes for this. Hold the first spoon, fork or chopstick full in your mouth for a few moments before you start to chew. Savor the texture and taste. Let your tongue give you all the information available, embrace the richness and nuances of the morsels. All of the wonderful things in life should be savored. When you savor an experience, or relationship in life it becomes memorable. Adding flavor and richness to life. The relationship you have with your food will determine the experiences you have in your body. Any relationship worth having is worth cherishing.

When you take time to relax and breathe before your meal it calms the mind, body and spirit. This will take you out of any aggressive, acidic mode you might be in. When you smell your food this changes your mood, awakens the body and the entire digestive system. Closing your eyes closes off the sense of sight and heightens the sense of smell. The olfactory glands connect the sense of smell to the sense of taste. The salivary glands become activated and begin to go to work. As we say, making the mouth water. That first bite should be an amount that covers less than half of the tongue. To truly be able to gather the senses, feel the texture and experience the taste. Never stuff the mouth and create a mechanical nightmare. As you slowly begin to chew let your food spread over the palate. Feel the change in texture as the particles are broken down as you chew and the wateriness as saliva is continually added. From time to time at various intervals put down the utensil and continue to savor your food throughout your meal. If you are with company discuss the nuances and differing aspects of the various dishes you are sharing. This is a very important step in showing yourself respect and appreciation. *A healthy relationship with healthy food is a foundational cornerstone for healthy relationships throughout your life, and a healthy mind, body and spirit.*

> Savoring is an art that only the most fervent chocolate lovers seem to really master.

Chapter 5

Vital Properties

Foods that have greater amounts of the following properties are what I consider to be Super Foods. These are the primary foods on the Foods and Frequency list. Including any of these foods in your **LIVE~IT** will improve your health. Having a good amount of them will add years of quality living to the average persons' life. The Vital Properties will enlighten you to how these foods benefit the body and why they are super. Knowing these properties will also help you determine for yourself the quality of what you eat. Rather than have someone else tell you what is good for you. Having a firm grasp of this information will allow you to do this for yourself, your family and group members. As you work with your team have discussions around this information. Begin immediately evaluating the nutritional and health values of everything you put into your mouth. *YOUR HEALTH IS YOUR RESPONSIBILITY.*

This chapter is to inform you in greater detail of the properties of the foods on the Foods and Frequency list. On the list, the properties will be given as single words, which correlate with the titles in this chapter, the exceptions being oxygen and water which have been discussed at length already in earlier chapters. Please be aware that each and every property listed on the Foods and Frequency List does not appear below. The most critical and easily explained properties are listed for you the reader to become knowledgeable without suffering information overload. The intent is to get you quickly on your way to better health and awareness.

Chlorophyll

Chlorophyll converts sunlight into food for plants through the process of photosynthesis. It is the blood of plants. It is nearly identical to human blood. Where hemoglobin has iron, chlorophyll has magnesium. Having magnesium in a good ratio to calcium gives chlorophyll its bone building and teeth recalcification ability. Unlike cow's milk, which is absent adequate magnesium and instead of building bone properly causes a calcium imbalance. Which creates problems the general public is not made aware of. If you want to build strong teeth and bones eating greens is the proper way to do it. Not by drinking the food of another animal's infant. Found predominantly in the leaves chlorophyll is extremely beneficial to the human body. It stimulates cell regeneration, is antioxidant, revitalizes the blood, boosts the immune system, destroys cancer cells and is so powerful; it's like liquid sunshine. Being the main source of the plants energetic resource allows the leaves of the plant to be combined with any other part of the plant for consumption.

Unlike the contrast between fruits that process quickly and roots that process slowly in the body and generally shouldn't be combined. Chlorophyll allows leaves to be eaten with any other part of the plant. Chlorophyll boosts the nutrient value of whatever else is consumed along with it. *This is why greens are such a vital part of a healthy* **LIVE~IT**, *and must be consumed on a daily basis.* As we look at the various types of greens in our normal eating pattern we actually leave out a lot of leaves that are also full of chlorophyll. Other cultures take full advantage of this bounty. We need to expand our pallet and begin to experience this richness also. Research has shown that Kale is the most nutrient dense greens on land; of those that have been analyzed. Kelp is the most nutrient dense food source from the oceans. Both are leaves that gather sunlight to create this abundance. These are a staple part of a good **LIVE~IT**.

Let's look at what other cultures show us. Other leaves that are abundant in chlorophyll and other nutrients are Amaranth (Calaloo), Grape, Okra, Sweet Potato and Yucca (Cassava) to name a few. We shouldn't take this extremely rich food source for granted. Especially since what we call food is becoming less and less nutritious. Setting us up for many diseases and conditions. Including all those that follow constipation and obesity.

We must increase our intake of leaves on a daily basis. Steamed is better than fully cooked, raw is better than steamed. The best way is to drink them in Smoothies. Cooking destroys enzymes thereby inhibiting the digestive process and diminishing the nutrient availability of what we might eat. Steaming softens the greens without totally destroying enzymes that aid digestion and the uptake of nutrients. Raw maintains all enzymes and nutrient vitality. However even for tender greens chewing adequately for the rupturing of the cellulose fiber to release nutrients is unlikely, if not impossible. To consume raw greens it is best that they are wilted or blended in a high-speed blender. For wilting tear the leaves into small pieces or pulse in a food processor with the S blade. Massage in lemon juice, sea salt and freshly crushed garlic (optional). After being wilted they are more chewable and digestible. To get the most nutrients from greens add them to Smoothies using a high-speed blender. Regular blenders have a problem blending the more fibrous leaves like kale and collards. For those blenders it is better to use tender greens such as amaranth (calaloo), beet, chard, lettuce, okra and spinach.

The other ultimate alternative is juicing. Juicing concentrates the nutrients. All juices should be diluted with 50% water and swished or held in the mouth for a few seconds to stimulate saliva production. Juicing removes fiber so you don't get the whole benefit of the greens consumption experience. However it is a powerful compliment to boost nutrients in the body. Particularly since most of us, like most of what we eat, are nutrient deficient. See chapter on juicing for more information.

I refer to blenders, juicers and food processors as mechanical chewers. They mechanically take care of that portion of the first part of the digestive process. Grinding food into small digestible particles. The second part is the addition of saliva. This happens in the chewing or swishing process. Given the overall condition of health in the general populace these mechanical chewers are becoming to nutrient consumption what fire was to the consumption of animal flesh.

> Having magnesium in a good ratio to calcium gives chlorophyll its bone building and teeth recalcification ability.

Enzymes

Enzymes are chemical substances within the body and raw foods. They are responsible for breaking down food molecules so nutrients are readily available for assimilation. The enzyme amylase has already been discussed in the chapter on Saliva and Chewing. This enzyme begins the process of breaking down carbohydrates. Food is then passed through the pharynx and esophagus, and into the stomach. There it is in contact with and acted upon by hydrochloric acid and the enzyme pepsin. Pepsin begins the digestion process for protein. Pancreatic enzymes along with enzymes and bile from the Liver are secreted into the Small Intestines to continue the break down of carbohydrates proteins, and fats. Nutrients are absorbed through the villi in the Small Intestines. Indigestible fiber and waste is transported to the Large Intestines for elimination. There are intestinal glands at the base of the villi that also secrete intestinal enzymes. Villi are finger like projections that cover the interior lining of the Small Intestines. When viewed up close villi look like plants on the seabed or a lush rainforest. They absorb nutrients and create vitamins, much like photosynthesis in plants, with the aid of good intestinal bacteria (flora). Some of the B vitamins are actually synthesized in small intestines, especially the all-important B_{12}.

The B vitamins are your energy vitamins and influence brain health. The production and absorption of these important vitamins is slowed or potentially halted when the intestines are coated with mucous. Constipation causes toxins and waste to buildup on the walls of the intestine also compounding this problem. Brain function becomes impaired and the energy level is low and the ability to focus is difficult. Some of these actions are seen as symptoms in Attention Deficit Disorders, Dementia and other brain disorders. Along with the slowing of metabolism, accompanying inactivity, and waste accumulation all contributing to Obesity and a host of diseases. Eating fresh raw fruits and vegetables ensure an ample supply of enzymes to optimize digestive function. I believe that's why the tradition of starting a meal out with a salad was started. Whenever possible eat raw, and when eating cooked food make sure to have a complement of something raw along with it.

Fiber

As we assess the wonders of the human body and the miraculous benefits of a wholesome **LIVE~IT** we have to marvel at fiber and the way it works. It sweeps and brushes the walls of the intestinal tract, binds with many damaging toxins, cells and particles to carry them out of the body. Like a sheriff throwing a bad guy out of town. The best source of fiber is fresh raw fruits and vegetables, including sea vegetables, nuts and seeds. There are two basic types of fiber: insoluble and soluble.

Insoluble fiber with its woody cellulose fibers does not dissolve in water and is the one that grabs the bad guys. Since it is insoluble it goes undigested. Maintaining its form allows it to brush away phlegm like mucous and other harmful matter from the walls of the intestines. Remember in high school Biology having to culture bacteria in a petri dish? Mucous and toxic waste accelerates the growth of harmful bacteria the same as the medium used in the petri dish. Removing them from the colon is a vital issue. Soluble fiber is then able to impart a slippery mucilaginous coating to ease the flow of fecal matter. The cellulose fibers of insoluble fiber holds water several times it weight, which causes bulking of fecal matter. This contributes to regularity by stimulating the empting of the colon. Processed so-called foods, meat and animal by-products devoid of fiber do not do this. Which is why many meat and cheese loving, vegetable loathing individuals go days without a bowel movement. The quality of what you eat and its health benefits can greatly be determined by the quality of your elimination. While sweeping the intestines of debris and mucus insoluble fiber also sweeps away some of the intestinal flora. Thereby lowering the conversion and absorption rate of some nutrients. This means that we must also maintain in our **LIVE~IT** consistent adding of probiotic and nutrient dense food sources. For that the Foods & Frequency chapter will provide you with a sound foundation.

Soluble fiber dissolves in water and is also fat-soluble. *Interesting word soluble; meaning able to dissolve into. When two liquids dissolve into one it's called a solution and we all know the word solution is a synonym for the word answer.* Insoluble fiber makes sure we are regular by increasing volume and shortening time between eliminations. Soluble fiber also holds water, but slows the process down a bit. If insoluble brushes through the intestinal tract too quickly much more nutrients and intestinal flora will be pulled out with it and, it could prove abrasive. Soluble fiber prevents this from happening by slowing down the process and adding its gelatinous form to both feces and the lining of the colon. In this manner it also slows the break down of carbohydrates and the absorption rate of glucose helping to regulate blood sugar levels. Simple logic: If a denatured low fiber empty carb **diet** can cause diabetes. A natural high fiber **LIVE~IT** loaded with plant protein and complex carbohydrates can prevent and reverse diabetes. Not only are fresh raw fruits and vegetables nonfattening, the soluble fiber they possess removes fat from the body, which in turn lowers bad cholesterol. If you add water to freshly ground flax seed and rub it between your fingers it is both sticky and slippery. These slimy, mucilaginous soluble fibers provide an **emollient quality**. Though this is a property of soluble fiber I feel it needs to be separated out, as a vital property in it's own right.

Emollient Quality: Foods high in this quality of soluble fiber actually soften tissue making it more pliable and supple. It's like internal lotion. This is very important because hardening of the skin tissue that makes up the organs and vessels is very dangerous. When hardened these organs and vessels become more pressurized, inflamed and susceptible to leaking, rupturing or splitting. The conditions that arise from this scenario are some of the most devastating and deadly. Heart dis-ease, so-called heart attacks, high blood pressure, strokes, and aneurisms top the list. Incorporating foods that have emollient quality is vital for youthful, and vibrant health. Free of these dangerous conditions that debilitate and drastically shorten life. Some of these foods are aloe vera, banana, flax seed, oats, okra, okra leaves, and sea vegetables. Foods that have a greater emollient quality are Super Foods, with enhanced healing ability. Though this is a general quality of soluble fiber those that possess greater emollient properties are extra special. As critical as leaves with their abundance of chlorophyll. Make sure to increase and maintain ample amounts of these in your **LIVE~IT**.

> ## It's like internal lotion

Fiber binds with harmful bacteria, cancer causing agents and other toxins and remove them from the body. A host of different cancers are prevented on an ongoing basis with a consistent high fiber **LIVE~IT**. We ingest through consumption, breathing and absorption through the skin cancer causing agents almost daily. So cancer cells are present at some point in all of us. Whether or not these grow, assemble and multiply depends on the internal environment of our bodies. Processed denatured so-called food, animal flesh and animal by products create the perfect environment for cancer and other diseases and conditions to flourish. A **LIVE~IT**, which includes whole raw fruits, veggies, and so on as described herein creates a pristine internal environment potentially free of toxic accumulation and cancerous growth. Regardless of your current health status or condition it is never too late to begin anew. Never too late to turn around any malady or ill, and quality fiber is a critical component in that effort.

Probiotics

Practically everyone knows what an antibiotic is. We take them to kill of harmful bacteria in the body that causes various infections and diseases. They also however kill off beneficial bacteria. As our general knowledge base grows we are becoming more and more familiar with the term probiotic. Some may use the term pre-biotic. Probiotic as the name implies are the opposite of antibiotics. Instead of killing bad bacteria they actually feed and culture good bacteria. The good bacteria are those in the small intestines that aid in the break down of food particles that otherwise might pass through without the body having access to their nutrients. Another function they perform is the creation of nutrients through a fermentation process. These crucial parts of the digestive process are extremely lacking in the ever-expanding bodies of today's population. Causing many who seem healthy and fit, or at least well fed, to suffer from undiagnosed malnutrition. These additional nutrients aren't extra but essential to the body's immune function and overall vitality.

The two primary means of getting probiotics into the body that the general public is made aware of is by eating yogurt and the lesser known taking acidophilus. The more natural way is to get them through real food. The manner that I suggest is by eating Yucca (Cassava) root, and Cabbage on a regular basis. Instead of eating Yucca as you would potatoes I suggest the Yucca be prepared in frozen ice cubes and added to smoothies, soups, steamed veggies, Popsicles, and raw food dishes. You do this by peeling the root slicing it thinly, bringing to a boil and simmering until it is translucent. Then blending with water until creamy and freezing in ice cube trays. Or, you could buy tapioca pearls instead. Tapioca is yucca. Make sure to buy them from a store where they are constantly restocked, to be sure they aren't old. The longer they sit on the shelf the more enzymes and nutrients are loss. Yucca has constituents that strengthen the intestinal flora. Cabbage is a practical miracle in itself, it boosts intestinal flora and aids their fermenting ability that builds on nutrients. One of the many reasons it should be a consistently regular part of your **LIVE~IT**. *These two foods should be at the core of everyone's food intake.*

> Probiotics culture good bacteria that create B vitamins.

Chapter 6

Foods and frequency

Aloe Vera – 2 or more ounces per week.
Vital Properties: anti cancer agent, astringent, enzymes, emollient, soluble fiber, tissue regenerator and water.

Apples, plums, peaches, pears, and other northern tree fruit – 2 or more daily.
Vital Properties: anti cancer properties, soluble and insoluble fiber, enzymes and water.

Avocado – 4 or more per week.
Vital Properties: anti cancer, soluble and insoluble fiber, enzymes, protein, oils and water.

Bananas – 1 or more per day.
Vital Properties: anti cancer, emollient, enzymes, soluble and insoluble fiber and water.

Beets – 2 or more per week eat greens also.
Vital Properties: anti cancer properties, blood builder, chlorophyll, enzymes, soluble and insoluble fiber and water.

Cabbage – red or green 1 or more per week: for every 50 pounds over 150 pounds body weight add ½ cabbage.
Vital Properties: anti cancer properties, chlorophyll, enzymes, lowers blood pressure, probiotic, soluble and insoluble fiber and water.

Cassava (Yucca) Root – 10 to 20 cubes weekly.
Vital Properties: enzymes, ideal probiotic, soluble and insoluble fiber and water.

Celery – 1 head or more per week.
Vital Properties: anti cancer properties, chlorophyll, enzymes, soluble and insoluble fiber and water.

Flaxseed - 2 or more ounces per week.
Vital Properties: anti cancer properties, bulking agent, chlorophyll, cholesterol balancer, emollient, enzymes, estrogen balancer, omega 3 oil, soluble and insoluble fiber and water.

Garlic – 8 or more cloves per week.
Vital Properties: nature's antibiotic, anti cancer, blood cleanser, cholesterol balancer, enzymes, lowers blood pressure, parasiticide, soluble and insoluble fiber and water.

Greens - 2 to 5 pounds weekly, have some daily.
Vital Properties: anti cancer properties, chlorophyll, enzymes, phytonutrients, protein soluble and insoluble fiber and water.

Green Smoothies – 4 to 7 days per week.
Vital Properties varies with ingredients. Check properties of each ingredient.

Kelp – 1 to 3 ounces dried kelp weekly, types of kelp: Carrageenan (Sea Moss), Dulse, Hijiki, Kombu, Laver, Nori, and Wakame.
Vital Properties: anti cancer properties, chlorophyll, emollient, enzymes, nutrient dense, soluble and insoluble fiber, water, (Sea Moss – nourishes the endocrine system) and (All others – rid the body of radiation.)

Lecithin – 2 to 3 tablespoons per week if liquid; twice that if granules.
Vital Properties: Fatty acid, lowers blood pressure, protects; nerves, vessels and brain, balances cholesterol, aids weight management and digestion.

Lemons – 4 or more per week.
Vital Properties: bioflavinoids, electrolytes, enzymes, phytonutrients, soluble and insoluble fiber and water.

Legumes (Peas and Beans) – 4 or more pounds per week.
Vital Properties: anti cancer properties, chlorophyll (when pods or sprouts are eaten), soluble and insoluble fiber, enzymes, protein and water.

Okra – ½ pound or more/week, grow your own eat the tender leaves and try red. Vital Properties: chlorophyll, emollient, enzymes, soluble and insoluble fiber and water.

Onion – 2 or more per week.
Vital Properties: antibiotic, anti cancer properties, blood cleanser, cholesterol balancer, enzymes, lowers blood pressure, soluble and insoluble fiber and water.

Mango – 4 or more per week, eat the skin also.
Vital Properties: most nutrient dense fruit, chlorophyll (when skin is eaten), enzymes, emollient, soluble and insoluble fiber and water.

Melons in season – 1 to 4 per week depending on the size, the Watermelon Flush is and excellent method of cleansing and jumpstarting your **LIVE~IT**.

Vital Properties: anticancer properties, aids weight loss, chlorophyll (when rind is juiced), enzymes, lowers blood pressure, lycopene, soluble and insoluble fiber, and water.

Molasses – 1 or more ounces per week.
Vital Properties: Iron, calcium and magnesium in good ratio, fights anemia, and aids digestion.

Papaya – 1 or more per week if large variety 2- 4 or more if small.
Vital Properties: papain – most powerful plant enzyme, major digestive aid, rids body of parasites (seeds), soluble and insoluble fiber, and water.

Pineapple – 1 or more per week.
Vital Properties: bromelain – second most powerful plant enzyme, digestive aid, eases joint pain, soluble and insoluble fiber, and water.

Rice – 2 to 3 pounds per week: eat black, brown or red rice never white, combine with beans to make the perfect protein.
Vital Properties: complex carbohydrate, protein, normalizes blood sugar and cholesterol, lysine, soluble and insoluble fiber, and water.

Soups – 3 to 7 days per week.
Vital Properties: varies with ingredients, enzymes, soluble and insoluble fiber and water.

Sprouts – 8 or more ounces per week.
Vital Properties: anti cancer properties, complex carbohydrates, enzymes, protein, soluble and insoluble fiber and water.

Stay away from all dairy products. If you use plant probiotics (Cabbage, Yucca) you don't need to use yogurt.

Substitutes for white sugar: Stevia, Gymnema Sylvestre, Agave Nectar, Aromatic Herbs.

Eat yams instead of white potatoes and know the difference between yams and Sweet Potatoes. Yams can be bought at many Ethnic Grocers. Yams have more complex carbohydrates, protein, quality fiber and nutrients while white potatoes like white flour have empty carbs.

Substitute nut milks or brown rice milk for animal milk; animal milk is for baby animals, if you wouldn't feed these animals human milk you shouldn't feed their milk to humans.

In 2008 I was consulted by a young mother whose 3 year old son had repeatedly been diagnosed as anemic and was constantly constipated. I suggested she give him Almond milk with a teaspoon of Molasses and tell him it was chocolate milk. She was to pour this on his cereal also. Almond is the closest to Mothers milk in nutritional values when comparing all milk beverages. Molasses has plenty of available iron; it is also a digestive aid as it has concentrated enzymes. I further suggested she feed him Carrot Slaw. Made by combining shredded carrots, raisins and vegetarian mayonnaise. After following both suggestions both conditions were cleared up within 2 weeks. The raisins and the carrots also have lots of available iron, fresh enzymes and fiber. She reported that he loved both of these new additions to his menu and constantly asked for more. This shows how knowing the benefits of real **FOOD** can make a major difference in life from the very beginning.

Chapter 7

Chlorophylled Smoothies

Blended Smoothies present us with the greatest opportunities for optimal health available. If you have the right mechanical chewer you can transform and optimize your health for the best possible outcome. There are a myriad of ingredients and near limitless combinations that can be blended to aid in creating a level of Internal Fitness that is pristine. *With smoothies we don't have to worry about counting calories or tedious measuring.* Just put in handfuls of what you like. Along with a few teaspoons and cubes of what the body needs. Add water and press a button or flip a switch. In a few seconds you can begin to drink your way to a whole new healthier, less toxic and waste filled, internally fit beautiful you. Raw organic nutrient dense fruits, berries, seeds and leaves will give the body what it needs. Allowing it to remove waste and toxins, rejuvenate internal organs and tissue, revitalize and oxygenate the blood and begin anew. This will contribute to a clearer mind and peaceful spirit.

When blended in a high-speed blender the cell membranes of the various ingredients are ruptured, making the nutrients more bio-available. This is a vital component of a high quality **LIVE~IT**. Without this increased bioavailability lots of vitamins and minerals would not be absorbed though the foods pass through our bodies. When you combine these nutrient packed foods on a molecular level in the manner suggested you create a synergistic mixture. This mixture will turbo charge your Internal Fitness and transform your life. I will list a number of key ingredients that I feel should be in nearly every Smoothie. Then a list of general ingredients to chose from just to get started. I will also give general guidelines to help making a good tasting highly nutritious Smoothie. Keep in mind these are according to my palate and yours is probably quite different. So feel free to experiment. I'm not big on recipes but very big on experimenting with the things I like and encourage you to do the same. Develop your Smoothies around these basic guidelines. I will help you create your own high quality **LIVE~IT**. You will never have to **diet**, or die from what you are eating. The key ingredient list is short and radically increases the uptake of the more bio-available nutrients. They are key in maintaining healthy tissue and effective functioning of the various systems, organs and glands, and the effective removal of waste and toxins from the body. While the key ingredient list is the inner core of all Smoothies the general ingredient list is a body of things tochoose from, but not to be limited to. Look for the ingredients in the Vital Properties chapter to learn why they are so crucial to Internal Fitness. Please make sure to keep a record of your own Smoothie recipes, and be sure to document your healthful transitions in your Healthy Transitions Journal. Remember this is your story and no one can tell it like you. I'm just a coach, here to train you briefly along the way.

Key Ingredients

Aloe Vera
Cinnamon
Flaxseed
Kale: or Calaloo (Amaranth leaves), Chard or Spinach if using regular blender
Lecithin
Papaya with skin and/or Pineapple
Yucca (Cassava) Cubes or Tapioca pearls
Water/Ice

General Ingredients

Anise
Banana
Beet Greens/Root
Berries, especially Blueberries
Celery
Coconut, Young or Jelly/Water/Milk
Cloves
Cucumber
Dates
Fennel

Fruit Juice Goji berries

Greens, any, but especially Kale

Green Beans

Lemon juice/zest

Mango: adding skin makes for a thicker mixture

Milk beverage; nut or grain not animal

Mint

Parsley

Sea Moss Cubes

Vegetable juice

Water/Ice

Natural Sugarless Sweeteners:

Anise

Basil

Cardamom

Cinnamon

Mint Leaves

Fennel

Vanilla Beans

Note: All sweet smelling aromatic herbs are natural sweeteners. But, without the sugar content, so use them liberally. Protein powder is not on the list. It is usually a milk by-product and as you read you will know I am not a fan of humans trying to grow up to be cows. A well-balanced **LIVE~IT** will provide the body with adequate slow released, and nourishing vegetable protein.

The following is the recipe for the Smoothie I specifically put together for my father. Some of the key ingredients have a specific effect on the blood sugar level to deal with Diabetes and the revitalizing of the Pancreas. It helped clear up his High Blood Pressure quickly because of the quality fiber and other constituents. I spoke with my father and got his ok to call it Edgar's Smoothie in his honor. The amounts described will yield 2 quarts of Smoothie enough for 2 pints to be drank twice a day for 2 days. So plan to make your Smoothie supply every other day so you can have it each and every day as you work toward better health and beyond. Being designed for use by Diabetics it can be greatly beneficial to all, especially those suffering from Obesity, Constipation, High Blood

Pressure, High Cholesterol, and related issues. This is the basic recipe I used when helping my Father in the summer of 2009. It is not a requirement that you have any of these issues to drink this smoothie; it is optimally beneficial to all.

Edgar's Smoothie

2 Bananas, Ripe (with spots on skin)

2 Oz Nopal Cactus Leaf

6-10 Green Beans

2 oz Aloe Vera Leaf

2-4 Kale leaves

2 oz Parsley

¼ - ½ Bitter Melon, seeds removed

½ cup Papaya and/or Pineapple

1 tsp Lecithin (liquid), 1 TBS if granules

2 Yucca (Cassava) Cubes

1 TBS Cinnamon Powder

3 TBS Flaxseed, Ground

Water

Wash all fresh vegetable and fruits. Aloe is easier to handle if frozen; do not cook Aloe. Peel Aloe, place pulp in blender. Carefully peel Cactus leaf, (can be boiled) avoid needles and be sure they are all removed; place in blender. Grind Flaxseed and Cinnamon in coffee grinder; pour into blender. Remove stems from Kale and add to blender. Peel Banana, remove seeds from Bitter Melon; add to blender. Add all other ingredients, add water to fill point. Start blending slowly increasing to highest speed and blend until smooth. Pour into quart or pint containers drink and refrigerate accordingly. Remember consistency is critical, drinking a pint twice a day is highly recommended. Anything less will be less effective and take longer to see a difference in your condition. In my experience most people are conditioned towards immediate gratification. If they don't see results in the short term they have a tendency to give up. Remember, you worked diligently for years to get in the state you are in. So let's be diligent now and give your body what it needs to turn this situation around as soon as possible.

Drink 1 pint half an hour before lunch and the other half an hour before dinner. This way it will curb your appetite and you won't feel the need to eat as much. What you're drinking is more nutritious than what you have been eating. So don't think that Smoothies ruin appetites. They nourish the body and satiate it's hunger for nutrients. If you are tuning in to the Art of Snacking, your Smoothie can be considered one of those snacks, or can be broken down into 8 ounce (4 servings/day) and be included with a snack of fruit, cabbage, soup, a sandwich, or chips and dip. Check your sugar level before each dosage of insulin, and make necessary adjustments. Keep a daily log and show it to your doctor upon your next visit, and don't be hesitant to make him or her aware of what you are doing. Remember what you are consuming in the Smoothie is **FOOD**; fuels and oxygenates optimally daily (real food). What we put into our bodies that wind up manifesting dis-ease and death for the most part is not truly food intended for the human body. Do not be fearful of this real food because it may be unfamiliar. When many of us were infants and were given the food that turns calves into cows by our misinformed parents it was foreign. But we accepted it because it was given with love and good intention. Well, though some of what's in this Smoothie is unfamiliar because of conditioning, it is truly not foreign to the body. It's recommended with love and awareness from years of gathering information that *will* maintain high quality health in the human body.

F.O.O.D.
Fuels & Oxygenates Optimally Daily.
Are you eating food or are you eating STUFF?

Chapter 8

Juicing

I stated earlier, juicers, blenders and food processors are great tools that add to a high quality **LIVE~IT**. They increase the bioavailability of the nutrients trapped in the insoluble fiber of many fruits, vegetables and leaves. These mechanical chewers speed our ability to make our bodies stronger and heal faster. Rupturing the cellulose fiber and exposing a far greater amount of nutrients feeds the body to enhance immune function. Taking advantage of these utensils gives us the opportunity to elevate the level of Internal Fitness.

Juicing concentrates the nutrients to give us a power packed healing beverage. Since the nutrients are concentrated in a fashion that is not what nature intended, we must dilute the juice. Fifty percent water is the general minimum. Since our bodies are designed to ingest these juices along with the fiber it is advisable to drink such juices with a snack or meal. Blended vegetable juices go great with chips and dip, salads, sandwiches, and wraps. As we eat smaller meals more regularly, to keep our metabolism going, juicing provides valuable nutrients and energy. Eating large meals and craving that full feeling, may give comfort but can lead to obesity and malnutrition. Eating a **diet** filled with processed denatured so-called food (Stuff) that is very low in nutrients causes the body to break down over time. A vibrant **LIVE~IT** has more nutrient dense foods and a greater percentage of raw foods with active enzymes. Juicing provides us with an enzyme and nutrient boost. This compensates for nutrient and enzyme deficient **diets** that allow for the build up of waste and toxins in the body. The increase of health boosting constituents slows the disease and aging process.

Juicing allows us to access nutrients from not only the part of the plants that we eat but also the parts of the plants we don't eat. It is a well-known fact that most of the nutrients in many fruits and vegetables are just below the skin. We routinely throw the skin of a large percentage of fruits and veggies away. Let's take pineapples for example. While we eat the flesh of the fruit the skin is tough and prickly so we wouldn't even attempt to eat it. However we know that it's filled with the powerful enzyme **bromelain** and that the skin is green with chlorophyll. Instead of throwing it away we can juice the skin and get at those extra nutrients. Also this makes it more economical as we get more from each pineapple we buy. Pineapple also has a reputation for easing joint and back pain.

I personally juice the skin of the pineapples I put in my daily Smoothie along with the lemon skin from my daily Lemon Water together. I do this by blending them in the high-speed blender with water. Then I strain this using paper towels and a Salad Spinner. The result is a bioflavinoid and enzyme concentrate that I add to water and sip throughout the day. I add this to stir fry dishes and other drinks too. It reminds me of a drink made in the Caribbean called Pine-Aid or Ginger-Pine. This similarity comes from the fact that Pine-Aid is made by soaking the skin of pineapples along with grated ginger overnight and sweetened with raw brown cane sugar or juice.

I've even experimented with making a plaster from the pulp leftover after juicing this combination and applying it to my back under a heating pad. The result was amazing. I immediately had greater range of motion practically no pain and felt invigorated. You will be able to read about natural home treatments such as this in one of my upcoming publications yet to be named. There are many ways to maximize the use of the whole true foods we get from the produce market or department. This, results in better nutrition and health, more economical use of our hard earned money, and a more youthful and vibrant natural lifestyle.

The following is a list of foods that make up my short list of nutrient dense foods I find more suitable for juicing. You don't have to limit yourself to this short list. Whatever fruits and veggies you juice the nutrients will be automatically concentrated and greatly beneficial to your health and vitality.

Foods for Juicing:

Apples
Beet Root/Greens
Carrot
Celery
Cucumber
Ginger

Green Beans

Greens

Lemon

Sweet Potato

Watermelon Rind

Keep in mind the Circadian Rhythm when consuming juices with food. Unlike water that dilutes digestive fluids and enzymes these juices enhance digestion, with their enzyme and nutritional abundance. However strictly fruit juices should not be consumed with vegetable meals, and strictly vegetable juices should not be consumed with fruit, as noted in the Circadian Rhythm and the Food Combining Chart. This can cause internal conflict, resulting in gas, poor digestion and malabsorption. Save the pulp from juicing. Some of it can be used to add to soups, make patties and my favorite and a staple of mine Carrot Salad. Don't forget its perfect for the compost pile. Here's my recipe for Carrot Salad. Its quite simple, basically prepared like tuna salad except using the leftover pulp from juicing carrots in place of tuna. Remember you don't have to be strict with the ingredients and amounts experiment to your heart and palates delight. Adding Yucca cubes increases digestibility and Sea Moss cubes and/or other seaweed increases nutritional content for an even greater health boost.

Carrot Salad:

Ingredients:

Pulp from juicing 2 lb carrots

½ cup carrot juice

¼ tsp dill

¼ tsp fennel

½ cup finely chopped onion

½ cup finely chopped celery

1 TBS finely chopped beetroot (optional)

¼ tsp sea salt

1 Yucca cube

1 Sea Moss cube

½ cup Vegetarian Mayonnaise

1 tsp Sesame Oil

1 freshly crushed clove garlic

> **Keep in mind the Circadian Rhythm when consuming juices with food.**

1/8 tsp black or other pepper of choice

1 TBS fresh squeezed lemon juice

¼ tsp grated lemon zest

Grind dill and fennel seeds in coffee grinder or crush with mortar and pestle. Combine all ingredients in mixing bowl and mix well. Makes about 24 oz of carrot salad. If you would like it to taste more like tuna salad add powdered seaweed. Hijiki is best for this. Be careful a little goes a long way and too much can be overpowering. Eat Carrot Salad the same as you would Tuna Salad, with chips or on a sandwich. My sandwich is Carrot Salad on organic 7-sprouted grain bread with avocado, lettuce, tomato, cucumber and fresh sprouts. If you are minimizing bread intake just use one slice topped with the same or wrap it all in the lettuce or other green leaf. Have a glass of refreshing juice with your sandwich for a thoroughly nutritious and filling snack. *Watch out, I'll have you happily contemplating the vegetarian lifestyle in your sleep.*

Chapter 9

Sprouting

Sprouts offer us another opportunity for optimizing the nutrient values in our **LIVE~IT**. Growing your own sprouts is a nutritional and economic boon. When we look at an individual sprout we are looking at a young plant in its infancy. As with all things and beings this is a magical stage of life. The life force is so new and vibrant with an abundance of energy. The nutritional components are set free from the seed through a metamorphosis that transforms from compressed energy that is now alive. The actual nutrients are multiplied exponentially. The oxygen and water content is more than just significant; it is abundant. Speaking of water many of us without knowing why experience mouth watering at the sight of spouts on a sandwich or atop of salad. That mouthwatering effect comes from the stimulation of digestive juices at the sight of high quality nutrients. The body's naturally aware when it is in the presence of food that is nutritionally satiating. A high quality **LIVE~IT** should always include sprouts.

The seed is nature's truest life preserver. After the harvest and the plant has died all that is left to maintain the continuity of its life and presence on the planet is the seed; its encapsulated offspring. This little capsule has in it all the genetic material to remake its parent plant. And just like an egg it also has storage of enough food to see it through the gestation (germination) and birthing (sprouting) process. When it goes through this magical transformation, like any other infant it is in its fastest growth stage. Also like other infants it has energy that abounds. The food stores are transformed and increase exponentially to fuel this rapid growth. The nutrients necessary to take it from a sprout, to a young seedling and beyond, are multiplied through the conversion of its starch content and the chelating of stored minerals. In the case of some seeds and certain nutrients the values increase as much as over a thousand percent with the general average being around fifteen percent.

This is great news for B vitamins, the energy vitamins and especially B_{12}, the brainpower vitamin, which is in limited supply in the nutrient deprived **diet**.

Once they break out of the seed and begin to grow they increase in size and weight. This is quite beneficial given the fact that you may start with 1 pound of seeds and wind up with 4 or more pounds of sprouts. Their economic value doesn't stop there. When you consider the vitamin and mineral content you definitely get a lot of bang for your buck. They stretch your dollars by diminishing the amount of other foods you would normally put on your plate that would cost lots more. Not only can they be put on sandwiches and salads, they add color and crunch to soups and other dishes. They don't have to be cooked so you save on energy costs and preparation time. The high water and both soluble and insoluble fiber content aid in their digestion. They are low in calories and cholesterol free. Since they are eaten raw they are loaded with enzymes. And, since the majority of all things sprouted are beans they lower not only blood pressure but also blood sugar levels. With their abundant nutrients they appease the appetite and leave the body nutritionally sated. Ending the constant desire to eat quantitatively as in the case of the nutrient deplete **diet** that has many stuffing their bodies. As I spoke of earlier the two most vital things our bodies need to sustain life is oxygen and water. Sprouts by volume provide an abundance of both.

I have been sprouting for years and find it to be very rewarding. It also gets me back to a sort of earthiness. It's like gardening in the kitchen and you don't need to till the soil or chase bugs and caterpillars or get bitten by a horde of mosquitoes. And for those who live in urban environs it's definitely a way to connect to your inner farmer. Organic seeds can be easily purchased online or from your local health food store. I prefer online, as I like to purchase in bulk, that way I get an even greater savings and I maintain an ample supply. I do however from time to time buy from the health food store. Beans bought from your local grocer can be sprouted if you can't find organic. If you're eating them anyway sprouting will still boost their overall nutritional value. For sprouts that are a little more exotic and unusual I like to shop for beans, grains and spices from other countries and cultures at ethnic grocers. I will give you the benefit of my experience and let you know my favorites. These are mainly my favorites because they sprout so easily, hold up pretty well, are generally higher in some nutrients and are tasty.

Sprouting Seeds:

Alfalfa
Black beans
Chickpeas
Fenugreek
Lentils
Sugar Peas

> The seed is
> nature's truest
> life preserver

I find that sprouting in trays or the plastic bowls that I have gotten from ordering takeout to be the easiest. Sprouting trays can be expensive and if you're not sprouting in good quantity can be wasteful. It's easy and more economical to just drill or poke holes in the bottom of the takeout bowl.

Making your Sprouter: Get two bowls of the same size and put as many holes about two millimeters in diameter and five millimeters apart as you can in the bottom of one of them. This bowl will contain sprouting seeds. The other bowl is for soaking and draining.

Sprouting Instructions: Soak your seeds overnight or about eight hours. Drain off water and rinse. Put seeds in bowl with the holes in the bottom and place that bowl inside the other one to catch excess water. Check second bowl for additional water over the next hour. Keep the lid on the bowl when not rinsing and draining. Rinse again every 8 hours. To maintain freshness and avoid molding or spoiling add one-teaspoon hydrogen peroxide to a pint of water and spray sprouts with this solution after rinsing. Rinse more often and pay closer attention during sprouting when the weather is hot. Near the end of sprouting place sprouts in direct sunlight to stimulate chlorophyll content for greater nutrient density.

Depending on the seed being sprouted, roots and shoots should emerge within the first two to three days. The list I gave earlier generally begins sprouting within a day or two tops. Rinse and spray for up to a week depending on the amount of growth you want then refrigerate and consume at will. As an organic fertilizer boost I put a few pieces of Kombu, Wakame, or Hijiki seaweed in the water that I soak the seeds in. This gives added vitamin and mineral content and increases growth rate.

Along with sprouting I love gardening. The gratification of watching a seedling burst through the earth and grow from day to day. Its leaves outstretched soaking up sunlight by day and literally reaching up toward the sky in anticipation of rain or dewfall. Harvesting freshly grown fruits and vegetables that; I myself have grown and sharing them with my young children through the years. Writing this book has been thus far such an experience. Encapsulating my knowledge between the pages sending it to fertile and eager minds with the anticipation of organic healthful new growth throughout the community.

As I have been writing this project has taken on a life of it's own. Stretching, reaching, growing and developing into a body of work that will undoubtedly pollinate the minds of many. Who in turn will cultivate their own healthy bodies, minds and spirits, and those of others they encounter and care about. It has also stirred new ideas in me, and a greater sense of giving. I don't mean giving in the conventional sense, but an openness of Spirit and my own ability to inspire others to do more and be more. Speaking of growing, giving and being unconventional. I've started growing the seeds of the avocadoes, lemons and mangoes I eat so many of. Soon I'll have enough to start a small orchard. But since I don't live in Florida right now I'll be content with potting them and giving them away. I encourage you to follow this example whether you give them away or not. Think about the millions of fruit seeds thrown into the trash daily. If you want to see a thing of true beauty, plant any of these three seeds and you will be utterly amazed.

A healthy **LIVE~IT** is filled with nutrient dense foods that satiate the body's need for quality nutrition on a continual basis. Consuming in this manner staves of hunger eliminates craving and prevents the stuffing of your body that causes obesity and the many ill issues that follow. At the core of such a lifestyle and food intake are streamline effective strategies and tools that economize value and energetic expense. Following the Circadian Rhythm, proper food combining, adequate water intake and chewing, juicing and other strategies mentioned in the Biodynamic Nutrition book, sprouting and consuming sprouts helps to create a regimen that puts you in an elite category. The category of the vibrant, youthful, energetic and internally fit: a shining example of human potential.

As you adopt these strategies and transform, your confidence that you are on the right path will abound. Those who bear witness will be astonished and even puzzled at how these simple strategies are so effective. The joy and happiness you will experience in your life will become infectious as you share these magnificent tidbits with all who will listen. Take pride in your efforts and know that I am proud of you and the earnestness of your journey. Drop me a line and let me know personally how you are doing; fabulous I'm sure.

> If you want to see true beauty plant
> an avocado, lemon or mango tree.

Chapter 10

Soups

I believe soups came about when our ancestors would gather whatever they could and literally throw it all into a pot of boiling water. I think that's where the term potluck eventually originated. It's been known as a poor man's meal. However, soups provide us with a wonderful culinary and healthy dining opportunity. I mentioned earlier how soup gives us a chance to get more water into our bodies. Having soup as part of a meal with a sandwich, or as a meal on it's own, gives us this opportunity without diluting digestive juices. It also reminds us what consistency food should be in general before swallowing. Soups also present us with a unique opportunity to clear out leftovers. I find that they are also a very economical way to go gourmet. Putting together a variety of colors, tastes and textures can bring out the chef in all of us. A nice warm bowl shared on a cold evening goes a long way to take the chill out of the air. A bowl of soup, like a nice sandwich or wrap is a great mini meal that fuels the metabolism and doesn't make us sluggish. Soups are versatile; they can be served as appetizers, main dishes, or snacks. They can be light broths or filled with ingredients of varying tastes and textures for a filling nutrient packed fair to top of an eventful day.

Soups should have ample water of course, at least one green vegetable, a protein; legume (peas or beans), and a complex carbohydrate (grain). Root vegetables are filling and great, winter squash/pumpkins add bright color and sweetness. Summer squashes/pumpkins and cucumber add color and aid weight loss. Savory herbs add flavor, aroma and maybe some heat. Coconut milk brightens and adds richness, while pineapple adds enzymes and sweetness; these both give a touch of gourmet and the exotic. Don't hesitate to be creative. If you've ever watched any gourmet chef shows you may have gotten hints. Notice that they mix vivid colors and an array of flavors to excite the eyes and ignite the palate. The way they use various colorful and flavorful foods with a splash of this and a dash of that proves that variety is the spice of culinary life.

There are a multitude of recipes for soups out there and many recipe books that list hundreds. So I'm not going to fill pages with recipes you can easily get elsewhere. The major recipe that is the reason for this book is the **O.N.E.** recipe mentioned in the introduction. You can go online and get many free recipes for soups, or do like our ancestors and throw whatever you have into the pot. I do something similar by opening the refrigerator and cabinet doors. I love to experiment and suggest you do the same. As long as you are using ingredients you like you'll be fine. The thing I love most about soup is that a recipe does not restrict you; you can just go for it. And, this is what I encourage you to do. Cook and live the soup of your life without restriction; **GO FOR IT**.

Chapter 11

The Art of Snacking

Who doesn't like a good snack? Whether it's a crisp apple, a sandwich to fill a gap between meals, or a bit of something sweet to quell that sweet tooth. There's nothing like a good snack. While we all may snack from time to time, snacks are a very important part of a good **LIVE~IT**. Generally snacking is done passively. If its done all the time that's not snacking that's grazing, not a good habit. I'm offering a different perspective on snacking. Snacking with a greater purpose. *We don't view them as such, but snacks are mini meals.* We can begin to take full advantage of this dynamic by planning high quality nutritious snacks at various intervals of the day. Snacking gives us an opportunity to develop portion control. When snacking, pay close attention to the Circadian Rhythm as well as Foods & Frequency. *Snacking on mini meals keeps the metabolism level and constant. As many Diabetics can attest it also keeps the blood sugar level in check.* Also nutrients are the preventative inoculants that when kept in our bodies continuously, boost immunity for consistent quality health.

After a workout for quick muscle recovery a snack of bean dip or hummus and organic corn chips is ideal. It provides carbohydrates to replace energy as well as complete protein to build muscle, replenish stores, and satisfies after workout cravings. Along with a drink of Lemon/Pineapple water to replace electrolytes, add enzymes and move waste and fat. On a hot summer day how about a delicious and cooling Popsicle. You can make this delicious treat more nourishing and healthful when you make your own and add Yucca and Sea Moss Cubes. Any fruit sorbet you make in your blender can be poured into Popsicle molds and frozen. Paying attention to the Circadian Rhythm you know these are especially good in the morning before 12 and half an hour before any other meal. If you have children this would be an ideal snack for them prior to mealtime in the afternoon or evening, especially if they are tipping the scale. You won't have to worry about the lack of nutrients because you made them from highly nutritious ingredients. Instead of the dye filled frozen sugar water from the grocer's freezer section. This is also an awesome way to cool down any time of day.

Think of the many different flavor combinations when using whole fruits. Banana-blueberry, mango-guava, pineapple-strawberry, cherry-grape, coconut-banana, mango-banana-coconut, mango-peach-coconut, cantaloupe-watermelon, coconut-banana-blueberry, the list is endless. I add coconut milk for creaminess, fatty acids and antiviral properties. To improve the nutritional value, health benefits and texture, add Yucca cubes, and Sea Moss (Carrageenan) cubes to your Popsicle mix. There are so many exotic fruits from other cultures and countries you can experiment with that you are sure to love. You can also enhance flavors with fresh vanilla beans, cinnamon, mint and many other natural flavorings. I remember growing up in Florida, elderly women in the community sold frozen lemon-aid and fruit juices in four ounce drink cups for a quarter. Yep, I said a quarter; this was back in the 60's and early 70's when a quarter was real money. All the children knew and loved these old ladies, and of course they made a little money to help make ends meet. And who's to say you won't find a niche and wind up with a line of your own gourmet Popsicles in some large, or small, grocery store freezer. At the very least you will be a hit with your children, nieces and nephews. You can be confident in the fact that you're sharing a delicious healthy treat and instilling good and healthy habits. Let them help you make the first few batches and see if you can stop them from making their own, they'll absolutely love this.

A new perspective Snacking with a greater purpose.

You don't have to stop with fruit though. I've lightly experimented with black bean dip, black rice and coconut milk sweetened with dates. My intent was to create a nutritionally balanced after dinner desert or light meal that was frozen because it was a near 100° day. I decided I needed something that I could have that I wouldn't have to heat up on the stove and would be filling, but just so. To my own surprise it came out pretty tasty and served the purpose. So well, I now eat one or two after a workout, bike ride or yard work to speed muscle recovery and to replenish. Once again notice the combination of ingredients; a protein, carbohydrate and fatty acids from the coconut. Perfect for the task at hand, pure culinary artistry. And of course while working and after, I have my Lemon/Pineapple water drink made from juicing the skins of the same to replenish electrolytes. *There's a popular sports drink that has a commercial out now that gives you this information while trying to sell their entire new line-up.* I've just given you a more natural way to do the same thing that is more economical and intellectually engaging. It will allow you to teach the youth in a manner that is both, tasty and much healthier. *You want to reread this entire chapter over and over to fully process and appreciate what a great gift you and your family are receiving.*

Making Yucca and Sea Moss Cubes:

Yucca (Cassava) Cubes: Peel Yucca root and cut into ½ or ¼ sections lengthwise, slice sections wafer thin and place all into large stainless steel or cast iron frying pan of boiling water. Make sure water is at least ¾ of an inch above Yucca. Cover and allow it to come to boil; turn down the heat to a simmer. Allow it to simmer until yucca becomes translucent. Pour off excess water and place in blender. Add water to 1 ½ to 2 inches above Yucca. Start blending slow for 2 seconds and gradually, but quickly increase to highest speed. Blend until it looks like pudding. It looks like pudding because that's what it is. You've just made tapioca pudding. Pour into Ice Cube trays and let freeze. A word of caution; don't continue to blend after it's ready, as it thickens quickly and could burn out your blender motor. Once Yucca is frozen remove from trays and store in freezer bag or container for future use.

Sea Moss Cubes: Thoroughly rinse; this may require rubbing vigorously between hands, 2 ounces of Sea Moss (Irish Moss). Soak overnight in a glass quart size or mayonnaise jar with spring or purified water and juice of half a lemon, with lid on. Pour off water (great for plants). Add fresh water to jar up to 1 inch from top of jar. Pour this water only, into 1 or 2 quart pot and bring to boil. Carefully pour water back into jar with Sea Moss and add juice of half a lemon and replace the lid. Let stand for up to an hour, you can cover if you'd like in order to retain heat. This will allow the Moss to soften without actually boiling it. *Pay close attention, what you're learning here is magical.* If you have a blender that has a carafe that has a removable base and blade assembly, that base can actually screw onto the quart size jar perfectly. After an hour remove the lid from the jar and replace it with the blade assembly and blender base. Secure it tightly and turn the jar upside down and place the base onto the blender. Yep you're going to blend the moss inside the jar. Blend until smooth. Remove jar from blender and let stand on the counter for about 15 to 20 minutes. This will allow the air bubbles to rise to the top. Skin off foam and replace lid. Shake gently as moss and water probably has begun to separate; but not enough to cause more bubbles. Pour into Ice Cube trays and let freeze. Once Sea Moss is frozen remove from trays and store in freezer bag or container for future use.

Yucca and Sea Moss cubes are invaluable, they can and should be added to nearly every dish or treat that you prepare. Yucca has saponins that strengthen intestinal flora and stimulate their growth, therefore is a natural Probiotic. Sea Moss literally feeds the Endocrine System. That's all of the glands in the body. Glands, after receiving messages from the brain secrete hormones. Hormones are chemicals that regulate vital functions and the body's ability to cope with stressors and day-to-day life as well as its emergencies. A weakened Endocrine System equals a weakened Immune System and leaves you susceptible to all kinds of diseases and conditions.

Adding one cube of Yucca and Sea Moss and ¼ tsp Lecithin to Popsicles, Carrot Salad, Smoothies, bean dip, or other dishes keeps them in your body continuously. Yucca is also a great thickener for gravies and sauces. When we are sick and are prescribed medicines they tell us to take a dose every 6 or 8 hours. This is to keep the medicine in our system continuously in order for the body to make a full recovery. It needs this for continuous rebuilding or fighting bacteria that is attacking it. They learned this many years ago from observing the fact that the body's needs have to be met continually in order to maintain good health. Adding these key ingredients to our **FOOD** preparation boosts it's nutritional value because it allows us to maintain a constant dosage of Probiotics and food for the Endocrine System. Lecithin is a fatty acid that's as vital for brain function as the Omega 3, 6, and 9. It keeps Cholesterol in check and deals with fat distribution in the body among other miraculous things.

Sample Day Long Snack (Mini-Meal) Plan:

6am Lemon water, room temperature

6:15 Apple, Banana, Peach, Pear, Mango 2-3 pieces of either or combination thereof or ½ small melon like cantaloupe.

7:00/7:30 Glass of water room temperature.

8:30/9:00 Chlorophylled Smoothie and or Popsicle.

11:00/11:30 Glass of water followed by one or two pieces of fruit or a handful of cut up veggies; carrot sticks, celery sticks, broccoli, green beans etc., or how about one of those exotic Popsicles or two.

12:00/1:00 Sandwich or wrap made with avocado or guacamole, carrot salad, lettuce, tomato and sprouts and/or Soup.

2:30/3:00 Glass of water.

3:30/4:00 Smoothie or organic corn chips with humus, salsa, guacamole or black bean dip. If you do the chips and dip drinking some of your freshly made juice would be great.

5:30/6:00 Small bowl of rice and beans, or soup, and small bowl of cabbage and/or other greens. Remember you must have greens every day and at least one entire head of cabbage per week.

8:00 and later Glass of water

If you feel you must have something after 7 pm make sure three hours has passed since your last meal and have fruit, or fruit sorbet or Popsicle in keeping with the Circadian Rhythm. Try just drinking water first though as you might just be thirsty.

It is scientific fact that when we eat smaller meals every 2-3 hours our metabolism keeps going. When we go for longer periods without food our metabolism shuts down and our bodies go into a storage mode. This goes back to how we were originally adapted to our environment. Remember according to science human kind began on the continent of Africa in a lush tropical environment with an abundance of food growing all around. There was no need for storing food as it was all around us. We were constantly on the move, rose and set with the sun. There was a harmony that existed between nature and us. We moved out of that environment and the world itself began to change. We eventually began to impact the world and cause greater and now more horrific change. Sometimes food became scarce and created a need for storage, both mechanically and in our bodies. In our bodies this adaptation required a slowing of the metabolism and an increase in the amount of time we were sedentary. This was necessary because the environments we found ourselves were harsher and yielded less foods suited for our original adaptation. So there were often times when humans had to either make great treks or stay put for longer periods of time. Food being scarce at times we had to eat animals just to survive. This was a short-term survival tactic that became a long-term habit.

> ## Say it with Me Mini
> ## Meals equal a Mini Me

With our great ingenuity we created strategies to deal with these issues. With the advent of commerce and eventual economic dependence these strategies and what they yielded have flourished. We are at a paradoxical space in time where with all of our modern transportation and storage capabilities we experience from relative to great abundance.

All the while we are physically more sedentary. Eating quantitatively as if we are in a time of shortage and have to horde food with every meal. Our lifestyles are such that we schedule meals far apart and gorge ourselves at nearly every meal. To the point our bodies can't move as they were designed and become massive storage centers for food that is not used as fuel. Added to that what we eat more often than not isn't real **FOOD** that fuels and nourishes the body, but **Stuff.**

Part of the mentality that has come out of this lifestyle is that if you eat a snack between these large meals we **spoil our appetite.** *If what we eat is more nourishing and satisfies the bodies hunger for nutrients we are not spoiling our appetite but fueling the body. Actually going along with nature's plan. Parents program their children against nature when they deny them nutritious snacks. Just so the children will hunger for the enormous meal they have purchased, or now less often, prepared.* They then load the plates with more than a child's body can handle and tell them to **clean their plates.** Children come here following nature. We change their natural breathing pattern, their natural eating patterns, their natural thinking and emotional patterns. Then the whole of society is in a quandary wondering what's wrong with the youth of today. And, why the children are obese and have diseases that are germane to folks much older who have abused their bodies for many years.

Mini-meals offer us an opportunity to get back to the way we were originally designed to eat and manage our metabolism. This is emerging into our awareness through various popular **diet** plans that are successful because they work with the way the body functions. Rather than a fad or some new age way of thinking or marketing, this is getting back to nature. Humankind is experiencing a rude awakening from a continuing and ever expanding nightmare. Well **The Art of Snacking** is neither rude nor nightmarish. It is in the African spirit of Sankofa, going back to retrieve from the past that which will carry us safely forward. Sankofa is often put into place when an individual, family or community is at a great crossroads and in need of great wisdom to overcome great challenge. **The Art of Snacking** is part of my Sankofa offering to humanity at this moment of great health crossroads and crisis.

Lecithin keeps Cholesterol in check, fortifies brain function, lowers Blood Pressure, eases constipation, and manages fat distribution throughout the entire body.

Chapter 12

Jumpstart

In the summer of 2009 I spent a week with my then 78-year-old father. Who in spite of his years is youthful and full of life without any outward appearance of illness. However he is a Diabetic and was also on High Blood Pressure medication. I asked him if he wanted me to help him change his condition. I asked him this because I know many become accustomed to life with illness and become uncomfortable with potential change particularly if the advice given is not from an MD. He said yes; I think just because I asked. But I was glad anyway, as I love my father dearly and don't want him to suffer. I had him do a semi Watermelon Flush. And I made Smoothies, soup with barley and vegetables, and steamed cabbage for him. Within 24-36 hours his blood sugar levels were lower, some in the normal range coming down from over 200.

After I left I figured he wouldn't keep up the regimen. To my surprise he continued on for most of the following month. The end of the week after I left he went to his doctor, who, to all of our surprise took him off his High Blood Pressure medication. Medication he had been on for 9 years. By the end of a month he said he had lost 15 pounds. (For the recipe for Edgar's Smoothie see Chapter 7). Having weighed between 190 and 200 pounds the majority of his adult life he was uncomfortable with being what he thought of as skinny. He also said the doctor told him he was loosing weight too fast and asked him what was he doing. My father told him that his son had him drinking these Smoothies. So he stopped drinking the Smoothies and regained the weight. He is back on the blood pressure pills and continues with his insulin injections. Needless to say I was disappointed by the U turn. However, and I say this with the utmost respect for my father, I was more surprised that he stuck with it as long as he did. And, achieved the results he did in such a short term. It let me know that my father had some confidence in me, that, he would even consider following my advice. Further it showed him and other members of my family how simple and practical changes can mean major differences in health and wellness.

I give you this illustration to let you know how small but dynamic changes can turn an unhealthy body into a healthier one and vice versa. The human body is extremely resilient. Giving it what it needs to maintain vitality at regular intervals will allow it to thrive. If my father approaching 80 years can experience these physical and health transformations in such a short-term after years of being besieged by two of today's most common and dangerous plagues think of what you can do. If you suffer from these or other typical issues of the day I urge you to consider this Jumpstart strategy to begin your turn around. Adapt them as quickly as you can. Though these are short term measures they begin your long term, life long healthy **LIVE~IT**. I personally want to see all humankind abandon the current day **DIET** and adopt a natural, healthful life sustaining **LIVE~IT**.

As you put these strategies to use, you, your resolve and what's available will determine the finer details. Don't get bogged down by becoming too meticulous about extreme details. Remember it is a process and the major key is consistency. If possible begin with the Watermelon Flush. Stay away from sugar, white flour products, meat and dairy as long as you can. Start each day with the Breath of Life Clinic and a glass of room temperature water with the juice of ½ a lemon (Lemon Water).

Watermelon Flush: Start on a weekend, as you will be making many trips to the bathroom. Start with 1 regular size watermelon 20lbs or so. Wash melon and cut in half. Place half in the frig for tomorrow and eat the other half the first morning. Remembering the Circadian Rhythm, fruit in the morning. Yes, I said half, no need to rush. Take your time cause this may take a while. If you have a very large watermelon you can start with ¼ of the melon. Also the seeds are edible, and like all melons, watermelons naturally have seeds. Again you may have to go with what is available and seedless is becoming more prevalent in stores, though you won't catch me buying one. Watermelon eaten alone will flush all the waterways of the body when eaten in good quantity as you are doing here. It will flush the tear ducts, the sinuses, the lymphatics, the kidneys, and the bladder. Along with flushing the urinary tract it will also flush the digestive tract. The time it will take to flush the digestive tract will be a bit longer if you are constipated, and if so to what extent. If you do not experience the flushing of the body as described you may want to eat more watermelon until you do.

This flush may trigger a healing crisis,

After eating the watermelon down to the rind, cut up the rind and juice it. This will yield a significant amount of juice. The pulp should be composted immediately. If you don't typically compost, spread it around the ground and mix it into the soil. The juice is to be consumed throughout the rest of the day. If you start with the watermelon flush early in the morning and you feel the need for something to eat before noon, that's a good time for a Smoothie. Instead of plain water you may use the watermelon rind juice when making your Smoothies.

This flush may trigger what is called a healing crisis. This is what occurs to many when they begin their journey on the road to wellness. You may get cold like symptoms because of the body having to deal with the rush of toxins being set loose as they are being flushed out. Since the digestive system is being flushed, what some may think is diarrhea is just the result of the large volume of water and accompanying pulp from the watermelon moving through. So do not be alarmed, once again, it is a process. Below is the basic jumpstart plan. If you have not read the information on the subjects listed go and read any segment that you may have questions about for clarity. Substitute Edgar's Smoothie for the Chlorophylled Smoothie if you are diabetic or hypertensive; or want to move even quicker toward ideal health and Internal Fitness.

Jumpstart Quickie

Day 1	Day 2	Day 3-7
Lemon Water	Repeat Day 1	The Art of Snacking
Watermelon Flush		
Chlorophylled Smoothie		
Soup		
Cabbage		
Chlorophylled Smoothie		

You may repeat this plan for another week or so. A jumpstart in any manner is a brief immersion. It will you allow to test the waters and get acquainted with a new way of doing things. It's your own fact-finding mission. Giving you the opportunity to gain experience and witness a different lifestyle from what you are accustomed. It lets you see how you can manage with a different set of parameters. With the strategies utilized here and the foods being consumed, you get to see that it is not so much different. In that these are common foods that most of us eat on a regular basis. You will gain knowledge both in your intellectual and physical awareness through reading and then doing. Learn about these foods and how to use their unique qualities to shift from mismanaging food to being empowered.

As you go through this one-week Jumpstart period truly notice the nuances in your movements. The way you breathe, your stress levels, whether you feel lighter or have a clearer mind. And take a good look at your grocery bill. Compare that with the one from the weeks gone past. Notice that it's really not expensive to eat healthily. From my own personal experience, I know for a fact it's a lot more expensive to load up on items in the grocery store that will slowly or quickly get you to a diseased state or condition. Be sure to make note of these tidbits in your Healthy Transitions Journal, and of course any physical changes.

This Jumpstart can be repeated at will. Play with it and see how long you can go with it. Just to test your own resolve. See if it will lull you passively into an entirely new, healthier lifestyle. Quite often when we see something as daunting or major change we recoil. Not even attempting to make an effort to try something new. My hope is that by learning about how the body works and using foods that are very familiar this won't be such a great challenge. Instead, something you can ease into. The Jumpstart is your opportunity to wade around a bit before you dive in fully. *Soooo......* **JUMP**.

Final Thoughts

I must stress one major point so it is not forgotten. Obesity, Diabetes, High Blood Pressure, High Cholesterol, Heart Attack, Stroke, Dementia, Alzheimer's, Glaucoma, Cancers of all kinds, AIDS, ADD, ADHD, Prostate and Fertility issues, Depression, and all modern plagues have a significant oxygen, nutrient, water or exercise deficiency at their core. All of these issues can be greatly improved upon, managed, if not totally eradicated by increasing, oxygen, nutrient, and water intake, and exercise. These are the greatest gifts you can give yourself. Give the body what it needs and it will heal itself. Do this beforehand and it will not get sick. *A whole and healthy you is the greatest gift you can give the world.*

Adopting the strategies in this book and others like it will allow you to become the type of role model you and others will be proud of. Know that we are always modeling our lifestyle to all that can see, hear, touch, taste and smell us. We make choices all day every day that present healthy or toxic examples of our own humanity. Like the late great King of Pop, Michael Jackson sang, we must all start with the person in the mirror, if we want to see change. Change in our relationships, home, family, community, and world.

Many times my quirky lifestyle has brought laughter and odd looks from my peers and family. The youngsters would frown at what I put on their plate that appeared unfamiliar. After being coaxed into trying whatever it was, more often than not that frown was turned into a smile of amazement. Followed by, "this tastes good, can I have some more?" One of my young nephews upset his mother when he repeated something I told him. He sat at the dinner table and asked if he could he could have some dead bird. Speaking of the chicken she had prepared. After asking him where he got that from, she promptly called me. Asking, "Why did I tell him that?" Of course I responded, "Because it's true, and children should know what they are eating." Present day lifestyle separates us from our awareness of our bodies, and what we put into them. I want to be an example of truth and awareness. If I am to be a role model willingly or unwillingly, my will is to model this. And of course it also boils down to the proverb, "practice what you preach." I don't want to tell someone do as I say not as I do. I know that the three principles of the natural learning process are first observation, then imitation, and finally adaptation. Knowing this I cannot lie to you, my own children or myself. Thinking any of us would do otherwise. Before we could comprehend language and words we began life learning this way, and will continue to learn this way, throughout life. Therefore, not only am I compelled to practice what I preach, but to seek out examples and role models that I wish to emulate, and be the person I want them to be. Bottom line I must **LIVE~IT.**

Learn, breathe, eat and enjoy life dynamically, be blessed.

BOOK

THREE

INTERNAL

FITNESS SERIES

Internal Fitness Series™

Table of Contents

Introduction

Book Three of the Trinity

Oxygen   **Nutrition**   **Exercise**

In order to truly master anything you must first learn the basics of what it is that you are attempting to master. After learning the basics you must practice them until you achieve a level of proficiency. Then you must continue your practice until you actually master the basics of your given endeavor. They are the fundamentals that make up the foundation upon which you will build. A strong foundation is necessary to build toward mastery. The breath is the most fundamental essence of life, physically and metaphysically. It is essential to physical, mental, spiritual development, and the **mastery of life itself.** Breathing improperly can cause one to have a very cumbersome life experience. Burdened with physical ailments and maladies, emotional and dramatic mental instability. And, lack of spiritual fulfillment. Mastering the breath will literally transform all of these issues. *Mastering the breath is a tuning in as well as a tune up for every aspect of your person.* As part of an engaging self-aware existence this is your opportunity to tune in and tune up through Internal Fitness™ and Breath Mastery, on your road to the **mastery of life.**

Having read the Breath Mastery book you should be very familiar with the Breath Mastery Technique (BMT), the Breath of Fire (BoF) and the Breath of Life Clinic (BoLC). It is important that you practice, to become thoroughly familiar and comfortable with these techniques before proceeding into this book. The various movements and short movement series utilize these breathing techniques to enhance the effectiveness of the movements. Throughout this book the abbreviations for these techniques will be used.

You will find that holding the position at the apex of any of the movements and applying any of these techniques will be more challenging and rewarding. This is an advanced application that will expedite your transformation, once you have become adept in your practice.

While I encourage you to challenge yourself I advise caution in attempting this application. If you decide you are ready for this start with moderation. Limiting the length of time or number of breaths during each use of either technique. The exercises in this book are in three different segments, lying, seated and standing. Begin at a pace that is comfortable for you and add as you build confidence and stamina. You can adjust the intensity of your workouts three ways.

By decreasing or increasing:

1. *The length of the breath.*

2. *The number of repetitions.*

3. *The amount of tension in a given muscle group.*

Whether working alone or with a group you should chart your progression as you adjust to higher levels. When working with a group and especially if you are a group leader, be mindful of where each member of the group is along their path of fitness. Encourage advancement but be gentle and remind all that pain and discomfort is not a goal. The mind should be still and except for the muscles being tensed the rest of the body should be relaxed. These are short but intense series of breaths and movements. Any exercise that you have done before is automatically intensified if you slow down the pace of the movement. When you add to that the BMT and BoF it can take you to the stratosphere.

Know also that these can also be supplemental exercises. When done as a warm up or in conjunction with other workouts they build stamina and endurance quickly. The breath is the key. These series will go a lot further than any other type of exercise you have done before in helping you learn and master your own body. Though they are intense they are very simple. With the greatest difficulty being the stilling of the mind. The Lying series will greatly enhance your ability in this direction. It was created for that purpose, and is a cornerstone. Since we all lye down at some point daily, it should be easy to make this series or a portion thereof a constant. As you do this daily you will find yourself enjoying and looking forward to this time for yourself or with your partner. This segment will allow you to advance your ability while lying still and doing the BMT, BoF, or Breath of Life Clinic. Your ability to meditate and experience its many benefits will also improve. Soon your mind will become still.

The Lying Knee Raises will get you accustomed to the movements in the least precarious position. This will begin the toning of the body and build your awareness of the movements. The Seated series is great for those of us who work at a desk or find the Standing series particularly challenging. This segment allows us opportunities rarely taken advantage of in today's need a gym to workout world. This portion also helps release tension during the workday and can do a lot to improve productivity. At moments of high stress you will find yourself automatically doing one or more of these exercises and clearing your mind. The Standing series is most challenging and particularly aid balancing both the mind and body. Being the most advanced portion of the overall series it will make you most aware of your body. You will find your self-doing your favorite of these movements often as you appreciate the transformation and strength development of both body and mind. *Your primary goal is Internal Fitness.*

This short book and series is a scaled down version of the Internal Fitness Series™ and book that will be available at a later date. Please document and share your story with others and if you'd like, I would love to hear from you by email. There will eventually be a DVD version. If your story is compelling and well documented, *don't hesitate to video record,* you might be chosen to be in the workout series or have your story featured.

Chapter 1

Breath Mastery

Within the various series and exercises in this book all movement is tied to the breath. Therefore we will begin with a refresher on the breathing techniques. First is the Breath Mastery Technique. Followed by the Breath of Fire. These two are combined in an alternating flow in the Breath of Life Clinic. This is a review but don't just read through, do the actual practice of each sequence as instructed. As you read you will immerse yourself in the flow. You will remember to take your time and be gentle with the flow of the breath and movement. Practicing the BMT, the BoF and finally completing the BoLC will prepare you for the movement series.

You will remember to become thoroughly relaxed as you begin with the BMT. Your mind will become still and all the muscles of the body will relax. As you continue on to the movements you will continue to be in a state of relaxation; only tensing the muscles or muscle groups being focused upon in the given movement. You will find that as you progress from one movement and series to the next your body will respond effortlessly. This will encourage your practice and you will become diligent, looking forward to your next practice session. Soon you will view this not as exercise but as a part of you. You will embrace this flow for the rest of your life. Now relax and let's begin to breathe.

Breath Mastery Technique:

- **Place tip of tongue to back of roof of mouth with the mouth closed.**

- **Inhale as slow as possible through nostrils; into the abdomen then the chest, feeling air on back of throat audibly making inhalation sound.**

- **Pause for 3 count.**

- **Release the tongue; gently relax jaw, opening mouth slightly. Exhale through mouth as slow as possible with an audible *haah* sound, as if you were fogging up a mirror; fully express the breath.**

- **Pause for 3 count; repeat sequence for a minimum of 5 breaths**

This breathing technique cannot be overdone. The more you practice the better and healthier will become. Consider your health and the overall benefits this will bring to your entire body as you practice. It is imperative that an increasing percentage of your breathing becomes deeper and fuller. This is an extremely passive yet very dynamic technique free of the risk of hyperventilation. You will practice it at your leisure when reading, watching television, at the movies, at your desk, and in the car, do it often.

Curling the tongue toward the back of the roof of the mouth lifts and expands the front of the windpipe. This allows for a fuller and deeper breath into the lower portion of the lungs. Expressing the breath slowly and gently with the *haah* sound engages the lower abdomen, allowing for greater expulsion of carbon dioxide. This creates more available space in the lungs for oxygen. Slowing the breath also creates a reaction in the body that increases the oxygen level in the blood. This is an extraordinary synergy with benefits that an attempt at description could not fully encompass. You have to experience it. *Remember to extend the exhalation as you progress. As you do this you will tone and strengthen the abdominal muscles dramatically. One quick caution, don't overdo the inhalation; do not strain the lungs.* You should be very relaxed at this point. Let's continue on with the Breath of Fire. Don't forget these are short rapid intense breaths.

Breath of Fire:

- **Place your hands on your abdomen so you can feel to make sure the breath is focused and into the abdomen throughout this exercise.**

- **While seated upright in a chair or in the Lotus Position (Indian style), place the tip of the tongue to the back of the roof of the mouth and inhale slowly into the nostrils.**

- **Keep mouth closed and rapidly exhale and inhale through the nostrils into abdomen as fast as you can for as many times as you can for 8-10 seconds.**

- Relax and breathe normally for a few breaths to regroup. Repeat inhalation; rapidly exhale and inhale for 8-10 seconds; relax.

- Lengthen intervals and practice time as your stamina builds.

That completes our review of the Breath Mastery Technique and the Breath of Fire. Keep the tip of the tongue at the roof of the mouth. Breathe normally as you take your time reading through the Breath of Life Clinic. This will allow your body to cool down, your mind to relax and refresh your memory of the sequence. Remember the sequence is four rounds of the BMT with three rounds of the BoF sandwiched between in an alternating flow. Once you have read through the entire sequence go back to the beginning and begin your practice. By now you should be adept enough that you don't need to put your hands on your abdomen to focus the breath. If you feel that closing your eyes will help you to relax and focus feel free to do so. As you flow through the BMT your mind will be still and your body will totally relax. You will go into a meditative state that will allow this stage of your practice to be effortless and infinitely familiar. You will remain relaxed and comfortable through the Knee Raises and get the knee higher while bending the opposite knee accordingly for greater balance. Proceed.

Breath of Life Clinic:

Alternate between Breath Mastery Technique (BMT), and Breath of Fire (BoF)

- **Complete 3-5 breaths utilizing BMT**

- **Pause for a 3 count**

- **Take one full inhalation**

- **Begin 8-10 seconds BoF**

- **Fully express the breath, pause for a 3 count**

- **Complete 3-5 breaths utilizing BMT**

- **Pause for a 3 count**

- **Take one full inhalation**

> The Breath of Life Clinic is designed to replicate the benefits of interval training; utilizing only the breath.

- Repeat 8-10 seconds BoF

- Fully express the breath, pause for a 3 count

- Repeat for 3-5 breaths utilizing BMT

- Pause for a 3 count

- Take one full inhalation

- Repeat 8-10 seconds B o F

- Fully express the breath, pause for a 3 count

- Repeat for 3–5 breaths utilizing BMT

5 Alternating Knee Raises per leg to be performed either seated or standing.

- Inhale using BMT

- While exhaling with the *haah* sound raise the left knee above the waste-line slowly with the breath; bend the right for greater balance if standing.

- Pause for 3 count then lower the leg as you inhale using BMT.

- Repeat on the right side.

- Repeat left, right sequence 3-5 times per leg.

Excellent. You will note that there is quite a bit of a difference in the way you feel in your body and level of confidence since we first started at the beginning of chapters 2 and 3 of Book One of the Trinity. I trust by now you have begun to see other changes in your body and spirit also. I sincerely want you to gain the great benefits that are offered here. Everything written in this book is for your growth. I have practiced it all. So it has all been proven to work, applying it, as I trust you have and will, will reward you with a healthful outcome that will be both our blessings.

Chapter 2

Internal Fitness Series

Lying

The various segments and sequences in this series will be done while lying on your back. This being the most relaxed position, will allow you to become accustomed to relaxing while engaging the entirety of the breathing apparatus. It will also allow you to become familiar with a portion of the Knee Raises. This is less precarious than doing them while standing and more comfortable than sitting. When doing the BoF back-to-back pause and breath normally for 5-10 seconds in between.

Lying Breath Sequence:
- **Lie on your back, legs fully extended; relax.**
- **Place hands either on your stomach, along side the body, straight out from the body or overhead; palms face upward or interlace fingers.**
- **Proceed with the BMT for 5 breaths; slow and extend each breath squeezing more at the end of each breath.**
- **Relax for 10 seconds; still the mind.**
- **Proceed with 2 rounds of BoF; 8 seconds; then 10 seconds.**
- **Relax for 20 seconds; still the mind.**
- **Proceed with BoLC for 5–8 minute session.**
- **Relax for 30 seconds. Segment concluded.**

Benefits: Takes you further along in the retraining of the breath, fully engages the lower abdomen strengthening the abdominal muscles. Calms the mind and lowers the blood pressure. Placing the hands perpendicular to the body and overhead opens and lifts the upper chest and shoulder region. Corrects slumped posture. These benefits are greater when done on the floor versus when done on the bed.

- Toning the abdominal muscles gently and intensely, with extreme efficiency and effectiveness, as we are doing here pulls them back into place, not allowing for distention. This process massages all of the organs in the abdominal cavity. Bringing the abdomen back in alignment limits the space for waste accumulation and the build up of toxins in the body.

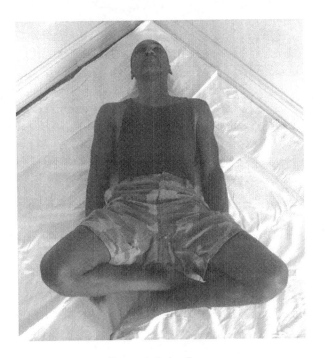

Figure 1: Lying Lotus

Lying Lotus:

This segment will be done as you lye on your back with legs spread and your feet crossed as in the traditional Lotus Pose. First with the left leg closest to the body then switch the positioning of the feet and repeat entire sequence. Whatever we do on one side we always do on the other to maintain balance throughout.

- Lie on your back, legs fully extended; relax.

- Grasp right foot with left hand over the ankle; place heel of foot against buttocks.

- Grasp left foot with right hand over the ankle; place it between your right foot and the body.

- Place hands either on your stomach, along side the body, straight out from the body or overhead; palms face upward or fingers interlaced.

- Proceed with the BMT for 5 breaths; relax, stilling the mind.

- Relax for 10 seconds.

- Proceed with the BoF for 8 seconds, then 10 seconds.

- Relax for 30 seconds.

- Proceed with Breath of Life Clinic for 5–8 minute session.

- Relax for 30 seconds.

- Grasp right foot with left hand over the ankle; place it between your left foot and the body.

- Repeat entire sequence as before with feet in this position. Relax for 30 seconds. Segment concluded.

Benefits: Takes you further along in the retraining of the breath, fully engages the lower abdomen strengthening the abdominal muscles. Calms the mind and lowers the blood pressure. Placing the hands perpendicular to the body and overhead opens and lifts the upper chest and shoulder region. Corrects slumped posture. Opens the hip and knee joints. Stretches the quads. Benefits are greater when done on the floor versus when done on the bed.

- Toning the abdominal muscles gently and intensely, with extreme efficiency and effectiveness, as we are doing here pulls them back in to place, not allowing for distention. This process massages all of the organs in the abdominal cavity. Bringing the abdomen back in alignment limits the space for waste accumulation and the build up of toxins in the body.

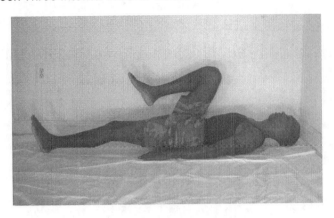

Figure 2: Lying Knee Raise

Lying Repetitive Knee Raise:

Note: During all Repetitive Knee Raise series of movements the foot should not touch the surface except when leg is extended in resting position.

- Lie on your back, legs fully extended; relax.

- Place hands along side the body.

- Begin the inhalation as with the BMT; all breaths to be executed using BMT.

- Upon exhalation raise the left knee slowly above the waste line as you make the *haah* sound. Pause for 3 count.

- Slowly with the inhalation lower the leg back to its original position.

- Repeat this Knee Raise for 3-5 breaths on the left and on final inhalation allow the leg to return to its original position.

- Upon exhalation raise the right knee slowly above the waste line as you make the *haah* sound. Pause for 3 count.

*Note: An alternative to this movement is the **Lying Alternating Knee Raise**. It is performed the same as the **Lying Repetitive Knee Raise** only alternating from leg to leg.*

Benefits: Takes you further along in the retraining of the breath, fully engages the lower abdomen. Strengthens the abdominal muscles, the lower back, thighs, and glutes. Calms the mind and lowers the blood pressure.

Gives great attention to the obliques, and hip flexors. Opens and lubricates the hip joints and stretches the quads. Benefits are greater when done on the floor versus when done on the bed.

- Toning the abdominal muscles gently and intensely, with extreme efficiency and effectiveness as we are doing here pulls them back in to place, not allowing for distention. This process massages all of the organs in the abdominal cavity. Bringing the abdomen back in alignment limits space for waste accumulation and the build up of toxins in the body.

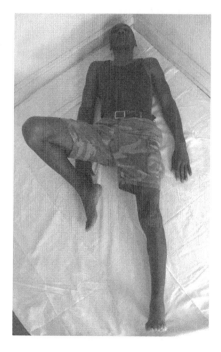

Figure 3: Side Knee Raise

Lying Side Knee Raise:

- **Lie on your back legs fully extended; relax.**

- **Place hands either on your stomach, straight out from the body or overhead; palms face upward or fingers interlaced.**

- **Begin the inhalation as with the BMT; all breaths to be executed using BMT.**

- Upon exhalation raise the left knee slowly to the side of the body above the waste line; keep the foot in contact with the floor as you make the *haah* sound. Pause for 3 count. Slowly with the inhalation lower the leg back to its original position.

- Upon exhalation raise the right knee slowly to the side of the body above the waste line; keep the foot in contact with the floor as you make the *haah* sound. Pause for 3 count.

- Slowly with the inhalation lower the leg back to its original position.

- Repeat this Knee Raise for 3-5 breaths on the right and on final inhalation allow the leg to return to its original extended position.

- Relax for 30 seconds. Segment concluded.

- Slowly with the inhalation lower the leg back to its original position.

- Repeat this alternating sequence for 3-5 breaths per leg; on final inhalation allow the leg to return to its original position.

- Relax for 30 seconds. Segment concluded.

Note: An alternative to this movement is the **Lying Repetitive Side Knee Raise.** *It is performed the same as the* **Lying Side Knee Raise** *only entire number of Knee Raises are performed first on one side then the other.*

Benefits: Takes you further along in the retraining of the breath, fully engages the lower abdomen. Strengthens the abdominal muscles, the lower back, thighs, and glutes. Calms the mind and lowers the blood pressure. Placing the hands straight out from he body and overhead opens and lifts the upper chest and shoulder region. Corrects slumped posture. Gives great attention to the obliques, and hip flexors. Opens and lubricates the hip joints and stretches the quads. Benefits are greater when done on the floor versus when done on the bed.

- Toning the abdominal muscles gently and intensely, with extreme efficiency and effectiveness as we are doing here pulls them back in to place, not allowing for distention. This process massages all of the organs in the abdominal cavity. Bringing the abdomen back in alignment limits space for waste accumulation and the build up of toxins in the body.

Lying Pointed Toe Knee Raise: see fig. 2 then fig. 6

- **Lie on your back, legs fully extended; relax.**

- **Place hands along side the body palms facing down.**

- **Begin the inhalation as with the BMT; all breaths to be executed using BMT.**

- **Upon exhalation raise the left knee slowly above the waste line as you make the *haah* sound.**

- **Slowly with the inhalation point the toe toward the sky extending the leg upward.**

- **Keeping the knee above the waste line lower the foot with the exhalation back to bent position.**

- **Repeat movement pointing the toe toward sky and lowering the foot for 3–5 breaths.**

- **Slowly with the inhalation lower the leg back to its original position.**

- **Upon exhalation raise the right knee slowly above the waste line as you make the *haah* sound.**

- **Slowly with the inhalation point the toe toward the sky extending the leg upward.**

- **Keeping the knee above the waste line lower the foot with the exhalation back to bent position.**

- **Repeat movement pointing the toe toward sky and lowering the foot for 3–5 breaths.**

- **Relax for 30 seconds. Segment concluded.**

Benefits: Takes you further along in the retraining of the breath, fully engages the lower abdomen. Strengthening the abdominal muscles, the lower back, thighs, and glutes. Calms the mind and lowers the blood pressure.

Pointing the toe isotones the muscles in the lower leg, and activates reflexology points in the foot.

- Toning the abdominal muscles gently and intensely, with extreme efficiency and effectiveness as we are doing here pulls them back in to place, not allowing for distention. This process massages all of the organs in the abdominal cavity. Bringing the abdomen back in alignment limits space for waste accumulation and the build up of toxins in the body.

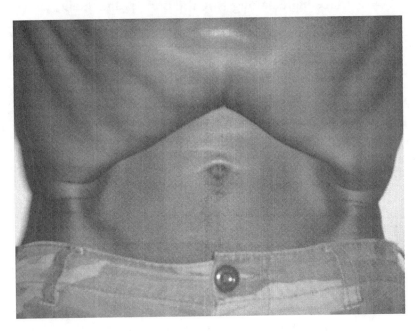

Figure 4: Drawing in Abdomen

Drawing In The Abdomen:

Be prepared to hold your breath. This segment is truly all about the abdominal region. The major component of this sequence is pulling the abdomen upward and inward after exhaling and holding the breath. Typically you would hold your breath after an inhalation. This is the exact opposite and only takes a moment to get used to. Also typically when holding your breath we don't try and move our abdomen. While this seems to be a bit unusual it is in the elite range when it comes to supercharging the bodies natural waste removal system and oxygenation of the blood.

- Lie on your back, legs fully extended; relax.

- Place hands along side the body.

- Begin the inhalation as with the BMT; all breaths to be executed using BMT.

- Exhale with the *haah* sound fully expressing breath as much as possible.

- Hold the breath. Without taking in air lift chest and pull in abdomen as if taking a breath.

- Fully relax abdomen.

- Inhale slowly.

- Exhale with the *haah* sound fully expressing breath as much as possible.

- Hold the breath.

- Without taking in air lift chest and pull in abdomen as if taking a breath.

- Relax abdomen and repeat previous step.

- Fully relax abdomen.

- Inhale slowly.

- Exhale with the *haah* sound fully expressing breath as much as possible.

- Hold the breath.

- Without taking in air lift chest and pull in abdomen as if taking a breath.

- Relax abdomen and repeat previous step twice more.

- Fully relax abdomen. Breath normally. Session concluded.

Benefits: Takes you further along in the retraining of the breath. Breathing techniques in general can increase oxygenation of the blood. This technique is ideal in that vein, diminishing potential free radical damage. Re-familiarizes and re-acclimates the abdomen to its natural positioning and activity. Revitalizes sluggish organs by bringing in greater oxygen and squeezing out more toxins.

- This is an advanced movement. It gives you the maximum front to back squeeze, upward pull and massage of the organs in the abdominal cavity and pelvic floor. It is very effective in milking toxins from the organs for efficient elimination from the body. Brings the abdomen back in alignment limiting space for waste accumulation and the build up of toxins in the body.

Chapter 3

Internal Fitness Series

Seated

The various segments and sequences in this series will be done while seated in your chair. It is designed in such a manner that will allow you to greatly improve Internal Fitness while watching television, at your desk or reclining on the porch, deck or beach. *Couch Potato, forget about it, this is Couch Fitness™*. All but the Seated Lunge can be done in any type of chair; this particular set of movements should not be attempted in an armchair or recliner. No matter what style of chair you use be very careful of your body positioning. Make sure you are balanced and set before you begin the movements. When doing the BoF back-to-back pause and breath normally for 5-10 seconds in between.

Seated Breath Sequence:

- **Sit comfortably with your back against the chair.**

- **Place hands on your thighs or arms of chair; relax.**

- **Proceed with the BMT for 5 breaths; slow and extend each breath squeezing more at the end of each breath.**

- **Relax for 10 seconds; still the mind.**

- **Proceed with 2 rounds of BoF; 8 seconds; then 10 seconds.**

- **Relax for 20 seconds; still the mind. Proceed with BoLC for 5–8 minute session.**

- **Relax for 30 seconds. Segment concluded.**

Benefits: Takes you further along in the retraining of the breath, fully engages the lower abdomen strengthening the abdominal muscles. Calms the mind and lowers the blood pressure. Massages, oxygenates and energizes organs in abdominal and pelvic regions.

- Toning the abdominal muscles gently and intensely, with extreme efficiency and effectiveness as we are doing here pulls them back in to place, not allowing for distention. This process massages all of the organs in the abdominal cavity. Binging the abdomen back in alignment limits space for waste accumulation and the build up of toxins in the body.

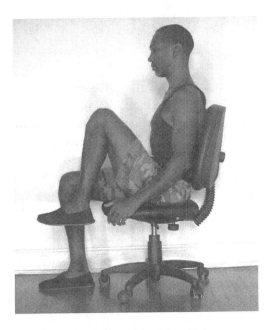

Figure 5: Repetitive Knee Raise

Seated Repetitive Knee Raise:

- **Sit comfortably with your back against the chair hands at your side; relax.**

- **Begin the inhalation as with the BMT; all breaths to be executed using BMT.**

- **Upon exhalation raise the left knee slowly above the waste line as you make the *haah* sound. Pause for 3 count.**

- Slowly with the inhalation lower the leg back to its original position.

- Repeat this Knee Raise for 3-5 breaths on the left and on final inhalation allow the leg to return to its original position.

- Upon exhalation raise the right knee slowly above the waste line as you make the *haah* sound. Pause for 3 count.

- Slowly with the inhalation lower the leg back to its original position.

- Repeat this Knee Raise for 3-5 breaths on the right and on final inhalation allow the leg to return to its original position.

- Relax for 30 seconds. Segment concluded.

Note: An alternative to this movement is the **Seated Alternating Knee Raise***. It's performed the same as the* **Seated Repetitive Knee Raise** *only alternating from leg to leg.*

Benefits: Takes you further along in the retraining of the breath, fully engages the lower abdomen strengthening the abdominal muscles, the lower back, thighs, and glutes. Calms the mind and lowers the blood pressure.

- Toning the abdominal muscles gently and intensely, with extreme efficiency and effectiveness as we are doing here pulls them back into place, not allowing for distention. This process massages all of the organs in the abdominal cavity. Bringing the abdomen back in alignment limits the space for waste accumulation and the build up of toxins in the body.

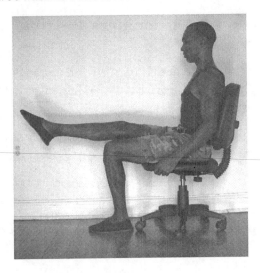

Figure6: Pointed Toe Knee Raise

Seated Pointed Toe Knee Raise:

- Sit comfortably with your back against the chair hands at your side; relax.

- Begin the inhalation as with the BMT; all breaths to be executed using BMT.

- Upon exhalation raise the left knee slowly above the waste line as you make the *haah* sound.

- Slowly with the inhalation point the toe forward extending the leg straight ahead.

- Keeping the knee above the waste line lower the foot with the exhalation back to bent position.

- Repeat movement pointing the toe forward and bringing it back for 3–5 breaths.

- Slowly with the inhalation lower the foot back to the floor.

- Upon exhalation raise the right knee slowly above the waste line as you make the *haah* sound.

- Slowly with the inhalation point the toe forward extending the leg straight ahead.

- **Keeping the knee above the waste line lower the foot with the exhalation back to bent position.**

- **Repeat movement pointing the toe forward and bringing it back for 3–5 breaths.**

- **Slowly with the inhalation lower the foot back to the floor.**

- **Relax for 30 seconds. Segment Concluded.**

Benefits: Takes you further along in the retraining of the breath, fully engages the lower abdomen. Strengthens the abdominal muscles, the lower back, thighs, and glutes. Calms the mind and lowers the blood pressure. Isotones and stretches the calves and the muscles in front of the legs. Activates the reflexology points in the ankle corresponding with the digestive and reproductive organs.

- Toning the abdominal muscles gently and intensely, with extreme efficiency and effectiveness as we are doing here pulls them back in to place, not allowing for distention. This process massages all of the organs in the abdominal cavity. Bringing the abdomen back in alignment limits the space for waste accumulation and the build up of toxins in the body.

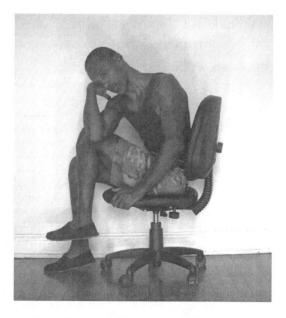

Figure 7: Seated Knee Raise With Crossover

Seated Alternating Knee Raise With Crossover:

In this movement you will raise the knee then the opposite arm gently placing the hand along side the face. Once the hand is in place you will then turn slightly and bend as you carry the elbow to the outside of the raised knee. This will all be done with the slow exhalation. Then while inhaling you will first lower the leg fully before returning the hand back along side the body and sitting upright.

- Sit comfortably with your back against the chair hands at your side; relax.

- Begin the inhalation as with the BMT; all breaths to be executed using BMT.

- Upon exhalation raise the left knee slowly above the waste line as you make the *haah* sound.

- Continue the exhalation, once the knee is as high as possible bring the right arm up; gently place the outside of the right hand on the right side of the face; turn the body gently as you lower the right elbow to the outside of the left knee.

- Upon completion of exhalation as you slowly inhale lower the left foot to the floor while keeping the right elbow in place until foot is firmly on the floor.

- Continuing with the same inhalation bring the body upright releasing the right hand back to the side.

- Begin slowly expressing the breath with the *haah* sound as you raise the right knee above the waste line.

- Once the knee is as high as possible bring the left arm up; gently place the outside of the left hand on the left side of the face; turn the body gently as you lower the left elbow to the outside of the right knee.

- Upon completion of exhalation as you slowly inhale lower the right foot to the floor while keeping the left elbow in place until foot is firmly on the floor.

- Continuing with the same inhalation bring the body upright releasing the left hand back to the side.

- **Repeat the movement and breath, alternating from leg to leg after each Knee Raise for 3-5 Knee Raises per leg.**

- **Return to relaxed position with your hands at the side of the body.**

Benefits: Takes you further along in the retraining of the breath, fully engages the lower abdomen. Strengthens the lower abdominal muscles, the lower back, thighs, and glutes. This particular advanced Knee Raise incorporates a bit of spinal twist with added benefits of opening the vertebrae in the middle and lower back. It also dramatically targets the obliques. Lowering the leg first allows for increased expansion of the lower portion of the lungs as the abdomen is automatically relaxed first. Allowing the diaphragm to drop with ease before the upper portions of the lungs fill up. As you experience this advanced Knee Raise you can begin to appreciate the beneficial effects of the earlier movements and the progressive and powerful nature of this full series. These simple exercises flow with the body's natural movement patterns (Kinesiology) and are designed for a streamlined, efficient and effective workout that doesn't require time away from day to day life at home or work.

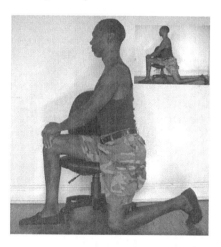

Figure 8: Seated Lunge

Seated Lunge:

Note: Should not be attempted in recliner or armchair.

- **Come half way to the front of your chair.**

- **Place hands firmly on the back of the seat of the chair and turn to the left.**

- Allow the right knee to drop toward the floor keeping the left foot firmly planted and the right leg perpendicular to the floor forming 90° angle.

- Make sure you are stable; place the right hand just above the left knee; place the left hand on top of the right hand; sit up tall.

- Begin the inhalation as with the BMT; all breaths to be executed using BMT.

- Slowly exhale with the *haah* sound; slide the right foot back along the floor.

- After the leg is fully extended begin the inhalation; slowly bring the right leg forward until thigh and knee are in direct alignment with the upper body.

- Repeat movement sliding the foot back and forth for 3-5 breaths.

- Place hands firmly on the seat of the chair and turn forward.

- Place hands firmly on the back of the seat of the chair and turn to the right.

- Allow the left knee to drop toward the floor keeping the right foot firmly planted and the right leg perpendicular to the floor forming 90° angle.

- Make sure you are stable; place the left hand just above the right knee; place the right hand on top of the left hand; sit up tall.

- Begin the inhalation as with the BMT; all breaths to be executed using BMT.

- Slowly exhale with the *haah* sound; slide the left foot back along the floor.

- After the leg is fully extended begin the inhalation; slowly bring the left leg forward until thigh and knee are in direct alignment with the upper body.

- **Repeat movement sliding the foot back and forth for 3-5 breaths.**

- **Place hands firmly on the back of the seat of the chair and turn forward.**

- **Slide back in your seat and relax for 30 seconds.**

Benefits: Takes you further along in the retraining of the breath. Fully engages the lower abdomen strengthening abdominal muscles. Calms the mind and lowers blood pressure. Opens hips, loosens tightness in front of pelvis, and strengthens muscles of the legs, glutes and lower back.

- Toning the abdominal muscles gently and intensely, with extreme efficiency and effectiveness as we are doing here pulls them back in to place, not allowing for distention. This process massages all of the organs in the abdominal cavity. Bringing the abdomen back in alignment limits space for waste accumulation and the build up of toxins in the body.

Drawing In The Abdomen: (see figure 4.)

Be prepared to hold your breath. This segment is truly all about the abdominal region. The major component of this sequence is pulling the abdomen upward and inward after exhaling and holding the breath. Typically you would hold your breath after an inhalation. This is the exact opposite and only takes a moment to get used to. Also typically when holding your breath we don't try and move our abdomen. While this seems to be a bit unusual it is in the elite range when it comes to supercharging the bodies natural waste removal system and oxygenation of the blood.

- **Sit with your back against the chair; hands on your thighs; relax.**

- **Begin the inhalation as with the BMT; all breaths to be executed using BMT.**

- **Exhale slowly with *haah* sound fully expressing breath as much as possible.**

- **Hold the breath.**

- **Without taking in air lift chest and pull in abdomen as if taking a breath.**
- **Fully relax abdomen.**
- **Inhale slowly.**
- **Exhale slowly with *haah* sound fully expressing breath as much as possible.**
- **Hold the breath.**
- **Without taking in air lift chest and pull in abdomen as if taking a breath.**
- **Relax abdomen and repeat previous step.**
- **Fully relax abdomen.**
- **Inhale slowly.**
- **Exhale slowly with *haah* sound fully expressing breath as much as possible.**
- **Hold the breath.**
- **Without taking in air lift chest and pull in abdomen as if taking a breath.**
- **Relax abdomen and repeat previous step twice more.**
- **Fully relax abdomen.**
- **Breathe normally. Segment concluded.**

Benefits: Takes you further along in the retraining of the breath. Breathing techniques in general can super oxygenate the blood; this technique is ideal in that vein, diminishing potential free radical damage. Re-familiarizes and re-acclimates the abdomen to its natural positioning and activity. Revitalizes sluggish organs by bringing in greater oxygen and squeezing out more toxins.

- This is an advanced movement. It gives you maximum front to back squeeze, upward pull and massages the organs in the abdominal cavity and pelvic floor. It is the most effective in milking toxins from the organs for efficient elimination. Brings the abdomen back in alignment limits the space for waste accumulation and build up of toxins in the body.

There has been a great effort in recent years by the exercise equipment industry to create equipment that will allow you to workout while watching television. Since, many of us spend an inordinate amount of time in front of the screen. A lot of this equipment has become an extension of the closet, being covered with clothes and such. That's if it makes it out of the closet or from under the bed. The Internal Fitness Seated Series requires no equipment. Therefore you have free reign to exercise at will in nearly any type of sitting environment. You can even have Seated Exercise Groups at your work place. With regular time allotted for everyone to join in.

I encourage you to bring this up at your next staff meeting, retreat or stress management session. This will compensate for those rainy days that you all can't get out for your regular walk. It will give a new dimension to the entire work environment and team dynamic. And for smokers instead of a smoke break filling the lungs with carcinogenic cigarette smoke. Take a breath break filling the lungs instead with good clean oxygen, and squeeze out some of that old smoke. Who knows all that good clean air might even cause you to quit that nasty habit. If it does you've got to let me and everyone else know. We're pulling for ya.

Many of us work at desks and sit for 8 hours or more per day. After such a long day a few who consider themselves fortunate trek to the gym. They work out, doing alternating cardio, strength, abs, and so on. The vast majority though, trek home to a large dinner the television and more sitting. While our eyes and fingers work away at viewing the screen, typing and remote clicking, the rest of the body just becomes burdened with waste accumulation from lack of movement. This Seated Internal Fitness Series is filled with simple movements that are the signature of the entire Internal Fitness Series. When done in conjunction with the Lying and Standing portions they will guarantee consistent attention to the breath and the abdominal region. This will ensure activation and supercharging of the bodies waste removal system. Think of it, between the Lying Internal Fitness Series and the Seated Internal Fitness Series you will be well on your way. On your way to a transformation you may have dreamed of but never thought possible. Take a good look at the cover of this book. No matter which of the shadowing silhouettes represents your current size and shape, believe it or not the fit body in the center *is you,* encapsulated in waste. It may take some time. But. By using the information given in the Biodynamic Nutrition Book along with the Breath Mastery and Internal Fitness Series consistently, you will achieve it.

Chapter 4

Internal Fitness Series

Standing

Ahh, back to the beginning, this is where I began originating this entire exercise series. It started with an analysis of various athletes and their movements. This was immediately after getting my Kemetic Yoga Teacher Certification. Initially I sought the input of my then Yoga partner and athlete, Sandrah. After a brief time I realized I needed to go further inward and began experimenting in isolation. I needed to slow everything down, literally. Tying the movements to the stillness of the mind and slowing the breath and the movements. Applying principles learned in my Chi Gong and Kemetic Yoga practice. Then and only then would I realize the true intensity and transformative power of these movements. As I learned then and you know by now that all transformation begins with stilling the mind and slowing down. . We must begin from an internal resting posture.

   I studied the movements of the fittest groups of athletes and the lifestyles of those who live the longest and healthiest lives on the planet. The fittest athletes seemed to be those who ran a lot; soccer (football) players, basketball players and track and field athletes, also gymnasts and martial artists. Those who lived the longest and healthiest lives lived mainly in hilly regions. Through my research I concluded that getting the knee above the waste line was a key movement in all of these groups. My research was validated when I was watching the only training video produced of Bruce Lee's Jeet Kune Do. Daniel Inasanto the only individual certified by Bruce himself to teach his style of martial art, stated on this video that the Mui Tai kick boxers were the fittest of all martial artist. And we all know that a major part of their training and one of their primary moves and strikes entails getting the knee up high in the air.

When we look at sit-ups that prized exercise for toning and strengthening the abdominal region, we see that it's a very unenlightened way of getting the knee above the waste line.

Welcome to the pain free no impact extremely effective Knee Raise. It simply can't be beat and will revolutionize fitness training for years to come. Let me make this perfectly clear there is fitness training and there is Internal Fitness training. This is Internal Fitness training at its ultimate and it is untouchable when it comes to removing waste toning and transforming and adding youthfulness and longevity to your life. When doing the BoF back-to-back, pause and breathe normally for 5-10 seconds in between.

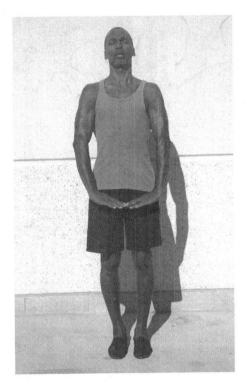

Figure 9: Resting Posture

Breath Sequence and Resting Posture:

- **Standing with feet slightly apart; knees slightly bent; hip slightly tucked hands in front of the body; arms extended downward palms facing floor; tips of middle fingers touching; elbows as straight as possible.**

- Proceed with the BMT for 5 breaths; slow and extend each breath squeezing more at the end of each breath.

- Relax for 10 seconds; still the mind.

- Proceed with 2 rounds of BoF; 8 seconds; then 10 seconds.

- Relax for 20 seconds; still the mind.

- Proceed with BoLC for 5–8 minute session.

- Relax for 30 seconds. Segment concluded.

- During movement sequence and at any point of high exertion or discomfort return to this position.

Benefits: Takes you further along the retraining of breathing process for optimal breath. Helps to relax, as the breath fills the lower portion of the thoracic cavity. The body relaxes, as in preparation for and throughout meditation. Isometrically tones arms, and stimulates reflexology points in wrist and hands corresponding to digestive and reproductive organs.

Repetitive Knee Raise: (see figure 5 pg.)

- From resting posture relax hands at side of body; extend left forward until the heel lines up with the toes of right foot; raise left foot no more than 1 inch off the floor.

- Begin the inhalation as with the BMT; all breaths to be executed using BMT.

- Make sure you have your balance; raise the left knee slowly as you make the *haah* sound; tuck the hip and round the lower back slightly as you raise the left knee above the waste line as high as possible; bend the right knee for greater balance.

- Slowly with the inhalation lower the foot back to the position aligned with the toes of the right foot still not touching the floor.

- Repeat this Knee Raise for 3–5 breaths on the left; on final inhalation allow the left foot to return to its original position along side the right foot.

- Shift your weight to the left foot; extend right forward until the heel lines up with the toes of left foot; raise right foot no more than 1 inch off the floor.

- Begin the inhalation as with the BMT; all breaths to be executed using BMT.

- Make sure you have your balance; raise the right knee slowly as you make the *haah* sound; tuck the hip and round the lower back slightly as you raise the right knee above the waste line as high as possible; bend the left knee for greater balance.

- Slowly with the inhalation lower the foot back to the position aligned with the toes of the left foot still not touching the floor.

- Repeat this Knee Raise for 3-5 breaths on the right; on final inhalation allow the right foot to return to its original position along side the left foot.

- Return to relaxed position with your hands at the side of the body and feet 2 to 3 inches apart.

Benefits: Takes you further along in the retraining of the breath, fully engages the lower abdomen. Strengthens the lower abdominal muscles, lower back, thighs, and buttocks. Begins the bodies adjusting and realigning by gently pushing to greater balance. Balancing postures and movements calibrate the left and right hemispheres of the brain. Enhancing clarity of thought and calmness of the mind.

- Toning abdominal muscles gently, but with extreme efficiency and effectiveness as we are doing here pulls them back in to place, not allowing for distention. This process massages all of the organs in the abdominal cavity. Bringing the abdomen back in alignment limits space for waste accumulation.

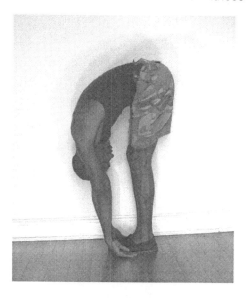

Figure 10: Forward Bend

Forward Bend With Hands Touching Floor

- **Begin the inhalation as with the BMT; all breaths to be executed using BMT.**

- **Coordinate all movement with the breath; slowly bend the body forward at the waist; exhale with the *haah* sound; reach for and touch the floor with your fingertips, knuckles, or palms, whichever can reach; bend at the knees if necessary.**

- **Stay relaxed during the movement. After fully expressing the breath, allow the inhalation of air to gently lift you as you rise back to the standing position.**

- **Repeat movement for 3-5 breaths; increase the straightening of the legs and reach gradually but gently with each repetition.**

Benefits: Increased expulsion from bending the body forward in this movement removes stale air and toxins from the recesses of the lungs. The contraction of the abdominal cavity squeezes the organs to hasten the removal of waste. The tendons and ligaments in the legs are gently stretched, as are the muscles of the lower back. An increase in range of motion and contributes to the progressive loosening of tightness in the body.

- The movements in this series are progressive with each movement gently preparing the body for those that follow. The latter exercises are more advanced. The preceding movements create openness and memory in the body that make them easier and more effective.

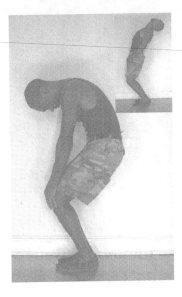

Figure: 11 Gentle Back Bend

Gentle Back Bend:

- **After completion of the Forward Bend With Hands Touching Floor, stand with the feet shoulder width apart; bend the knees to about a 30° to 35° angle; tuck the hip and curl the body forward with the hands resting on the kneecaps.**

- **Relax the neck and shoulders; allow the head to gently fall forward half way.**

- **Slowly inhale allowing the influx of air to lift your upper torso; lean back keeping the hands in front of you; rise to the point that the heel of the hands are resting at the top of the upper thighs.**

- **Project the hips forward lifting the chest; allow the head to go back about half way.**

- **Upon full inhalation relax and begin your exhalation remembering the *haah* sound; gently bring the body back to the starting position; slowly bring the head forward sinking in the chest contracting the abdomen.**

- **Slide the hands back to where they were with the palms over the kneecaps; the back should be curved forming a C not V and the knees still bent.**

- **Repeat movement for 3-5 breaths increasing the amount of time of each inhalation and exhalation to continue the development of increased breathing capacity.**

- **Return to relaxed position with your hands at the side of the body and feet 2 to 3 inches apart.**

Benefits: Gently opens the area of the upper chest while flexing the full length of the spine. Flexing the spine in this manner opens the vertebrae, front and back, stimulating the central nervous system. Brings fluid to spine and moves lymph throughout the body.

- Sedentary lifestyles especially one where there is a lot of sitting and a body that carries a large amount of waste puts a lot of pressure on the spine. Over time the lower vertebrae can become compressed and even fused. This contributes to a lot of low back pain and issues. Flexing the spine and opening space between the vertebrae throughout life is the ideal way to avoid these issues.

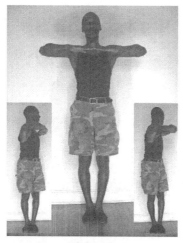

Figure 12: Upper Body Twist

Upper Body Twist:

Like the Crossover Knee Raises this segment is a combination movement that is segmented. The three segments are performed in one breath. First you turn the body with head and arms moving together. Then the arms stay in place as the head continues to move then the head stays in place as the arms continue till the end of exhalation. After the full exhalation the movements are reversed with the slow inhalation. Arms then head then both together in the turn returning to original position. Flow with the breath and relax. When the mind is calm and relaxed this is a gentle and meditative flow.

- **As you slowly inhale the body upright stand straight with the feet slightly apart; bring the tips of the middle fingers together; palms facing down toward the floor until the hands are in front of the throat; the arms are extended elbows out parallel to the floor.**

- **Slowly exhale with the *haah* sound; turn the upper body to the left keeping the eyes and nose directly in line with the tips of middle fingers.**

- **Once you're facing directly over the left hip hold the arms there; continue rotating the head to the left until the nose lines up with the left elbow.**

- **Continuing with the exhalation push the left elbow as far back as you can in the same direction.**

- **Once you have fully exhausted the breath and have gone as far as you can in the twist begin your inhalation; slowly rotate your body back to center.**

- **Bring the left elbow back in line with the nose then the nose back in line with the fingertips and left hip; continue until you are facing forward.**

- **Slowly exhale with the *haah* sound; turn the upper body to the right keeping the eyes and nose directly in line with the tips of middle fingers.**

- **Once you're facing directly over the right hip hold the arms there; continue rotating the head to the right until the nose lines up with the right elbow.**

- Continuing with the exhalation push the right elbow as far back as you can in the same direction.

- Once you have fully exhausted the breath and have gone as far as you can in the twist begin your inhalation and slowly rotate your body back to center.

- Bring the right elbow back in line with the nose then the nose back in line with the fingertips and right hip; continue until you are facing forward.

- Continue with this process until you have rotated 3-5 times to the left and right.

- Though this set of movements are segmented it is still one continuous flow without stopping except briefly at the backend of the twist and facing forward.

- Return to relaxed position with your hands at the side of the body and feet 2 to 3 inches apart.

Benefits: Twists the spine in both directions from side to side, particularly the middle and upper portion. Opens space between each vertebra. Brings fluid into the area, providing lubrication to the spinal column. Isotones the obliques, the muscles of the neck and shoulders, upper and middle back.

- Sedentary lifestyles especially one where there is a lot of sitting and a body that carries a large amount of waste compresses the spine. Over time the lower vertebrae can become compressed and even fused. This contributes to a lot to inflexibility and low back pain and issues. Flexing the spine and opening space between the vertebrae throughout life is an ideal way to avoid some of these issues.

Alternating Knee Raise: (see figure 5 pg.)

- Begin the inhalation as with the BMT; all breaths to be executed using BMT.

- Making sure you have your balance; raise the left knee slowly as you make the *haah* sound; tuck the hip and round the lower back slightly as you bend the right knee gently; raise the left knee above the waste line as high as possible.

- Slowly with the inhalation lower the foot back to the floor.

- Once the left foot is on the floor immediately shift the weight of the body to the left foot; with the inhalation slowly raise the right knee above the waste line.

- Remember to tuck the hip and round the lower back; bend the left knee gently as you emphasize the *haah* sound.

- Lower the right foot as you gently inhale, shift the weight to the right foot and continue with the left as before.

- Repeat the breath and movement; alternating from leg to leg after each Knee Raise for 3-5 Knee Raises per leg.

- Return to relaxed position with your hands at the side of the body and feet 6 inches apart.

Benefits: Takes you further along in the retraining of the breath, fully engages the lower abdomen. Strengthens lower abdominal muscles, the lower back, thighs, and buttocks. Extends the bodies adjusting and realigning gently pushing toward greater balance. Alternating immediately from leg to leg increases the balancing ability for greater equilibrium. Balancing postures and movements calibrate the left and right hemispheres of the brain. Enhances clarity of thought and calmness of the mind.

- Toning the abdominal muscles gently, but with extreme efficiency and effectiveness as we are doing here pulls them back into place, not allowing for distention. This process massages all of the organs in the abdominal cavity. Bringing the abdomen back in alignment limits space for waste accumulation.

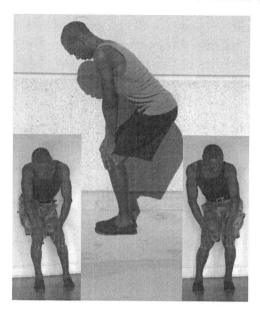

Figure 13: Quarter Circle Hip Rotation

Quarter Circle Hip Rotation:

- Spread feet shoulder width apart; place hands on knees; bend knees until legs are at a 35-degree angle.

- Begin the inhalation as with the BMT, all breaths to be executed using BMT; project hip and buttocks back.

- Exhale slowly with the *haah* sound; rotate the hip slowly toward the left in a circular motion 90° reaching the point that would be one quarter of a full circle squeezing out full breath.

- After full expulsion, inhale slowly; slowly return the hips back to center.

- After returning to center slowly exhale; emphasize the *haah* sound as you rotate the hip slowly toward the right in a circular motion 90° reaching the point that would be one quarter of a full circle.

- After full expulsion, inhale slowly; slowly return the hips back to center.

- **Repeat sequence side to side for 3–5 breaths on each side. During this movement be careful not to swing the hips or swivel the knees or head from left to right, all movement should be deliberate and focused in the lower back and hips only.**

- **Return to relaxed position with your hands at the side of the body and feet 6 inches apart.**

Benefits: Opens the vertebrae in the lumbar region, swivels the sacrum, bringing energy in the abdominal cavity and the reproductive organs in particular. Tones and strengthens the abdominal muscles with a great amount of attention given to the obliques. Can also alleviate lower back pain.

- Spinal twists and back bends help realign the spine and may gently correct some curvatures over time.

Drawing In The Abdomen: (see figure 4)

Be prepared to hold your breath. This segment is truly all about the abdominal region. The major component of this sequence is pulling the abdomen upward and inward after exhaling and holding the breath. Typically you would hold your breath after an inhalation. This is the exact opposite and only takes a moment to get used to. Also typically when holding your breath we don't try and move our abdomen. While this seems to be a bit unusual it is in the elite range when it comes to supercharging the bodies natural waste removal system and oxygenation of the blood.

- **Spread feet shoulder width apart.**

- **As you exhale slowly with the *haah* sound bend the knees to about a 30° to 35° degree angle; tuck the hip and curl the body forward with the hands resting on the kneecaps.**

- **Relax the neck and shoulders; allow the head to gently fall forward half way.**

- **Fully express the breath; hold the breath and lift in the chest as you would if you were inhaling slowly but deeply. This will cause the abdomen to be drawn in and upward.**

- **Do this three times; relax the abdomen and inhale slowly.**

- **Repeat the exhalation and holding of the breath and drawing in of the abdomen sequence three times pausing in between to catch your breath if necessary.**

- **Return to the relaxed position with hands at the side of the body.**

Benefits: In the league of the ultimate breath retraining movements. Calms and brings confidence to the breathing apparatus. Helps hyper oxygenate the blood without risking hyperventilation. Pulls in the abs and massages the organs in the abdominal and thoracic cavity as well as the pelvic floor. Limits space for waste increasing its removal in increased volume dispelling gas as well. This movement is key to this program.

- After having practiced this move both lying and seated you should have a level of proficiency that will allow comfort doing this movement while standing. Creating greater Internal Fitness maintains youthful vitality.

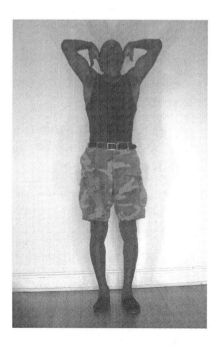

Figure 14: Fountain of Youth

Fountain of Youth:

- Stand with your feet 6 to 8 inches apart; exhale slowly with the *haah* sound; slowly bend forward at the waist; allow your head to hang freely; bring the fingertips to the floor at the insteps of the feet.

- Coordinate the breath with the movement; slowly inhale and rise up tracing the fingers gently along the inside of the legs and thighs over the front of the body along side the neck and over the back of the ears.

- As the hands come over the ears begin your exhalation with the *haah* sound; trace the backs of the fingers along the outside of the face and down the outside of the body.

- Bend forward at the waist until you reach the ankles; let the hands float away from the body outwardly.

- Bring the hands with the fingertips back along side the insteps and repeat the movements for 3-5 breaths.

- Upon completion of the final exhalation inhale the body up stretching the arms directly out at the sides.

- Continue carrying them up until the palms come together overhead.

- Exhale gently through the nostrils as you bring the hands down still with the palms together until they are resting in front of the sternum.

- Allow the head to drop forward and focus the eyes on the tips of the middle fingers with a tight but gentle squint.

- Continue to focus on the fingertips as you continue to breath through the nostrils, tongue at the roof of the mouth for 3 minutes.

- You have now concluded the Internal Fitness & Breath Mastery Standing Series.

Peace And Blessings

Benefits: Like fountain waters surging upward until gravity compels it to fall cascading out and down back to earth. Renewed energy from the earth is drawn upward through the body's center and stagnant energy cascades downward outside the body returning to earth for rejuvenation. Tracing the body stimulates the energy meridians along the body and resonate the body's electromagnetic field subtly increasing vitality. All of the blood in the entire body courses through the eyes every three minutes. Holding the hands in the Prayer Position at the end bathes all the blood with energy from the heart. This final gentle brush followed by the 3-minute meditation relaxes the body as its reenergizes and brings about inner peace.

- This series of movements is in the zero impact range. There's no jarring, or pounding. No micro fracturing of bone, tearing muscle from bone or wearing away of cartilage. Instead there is toning of muscle, natural lubrication of joints, massaging of organs increased flow of oxygen in the entire body. Especially in the organs and glands. When practiced regularly one can achieve a rhythmic flow that will have you in a calm and meditative state throughout as when practicing Yoga, Tai Chi, or Chi Gong.

Final Thoughts

As I have traveled life's road on this particular journey I have as always been reflective. Two memories of poignant moments in my life have stood out during this process. When everyone in the classroom was asked by the teacher in 3rd or 4th grade, "What do you want to be when you grow up?" The first thing that came out of my mouth without even thinking was, "A Man." I don't think I was being obnoxious, but of course some of my classmates thought I was just plain stupid. This memory has presented itself several times in life. Mainly when I am either at a crossroads or in the process of doing something very gratifying. In this case it's both.

You see upon reflection of that statement made in my youth, I've tried to access what means to be a Man. To be a Man is to be responsible, practical and true. True to one's self and others, especially family. Responsible enough to be considerate, and share with others those gifts that you have been given that help in time of need. Practical in the way you use resources and manage your affairs. These are simple measures. I have found that the simple things are what really matter on this journey. When things seem to be really complex and overwhelming I am mindful that complexities are nothing more than a series of simplicities strung together. The practicality of manhood and its foundational rootedness is what I believe stirred in me that day long ago. Without this grounding the quality of whatever I may have become would not have been true. That trueness has carried me through and I hope is reflected in this work and the path I am currently on.

The second memory is of when I was 17½ and preparing to leave home for the Army. I was at a shopping mall passing a table that was filled with wallets in front of a store. I can't recall if I had owned a real wallet up until then. I certainly hadn't had anything to put in one before then. As I looked over the wallets trying to make a selection one in particular caught my eye. It had an engraving on it. It read, " Mathew 5:16 Let your light so shine before men, that they may see your good works, and glorify your father which is in heaven." I hope and pray that this will come to pass with this book and the rest of my journey.

Oxygen Nutrition Exercise the holy trinity of internal fitness and eternal health.

Breathe, Eat and Exercise your right to be healthy.

APPENDIX

Reading List

African Holistic Health
By Llaila O. Afrika

Ancient Future
By Wayne B. Chandler

Between Heaven and Earth
Harriet Beinfield, L.Ac. and Efrem Korngold, L.Ac., O.M.D.

Energy Medicine
Donna Eden with David Feinstein

Green for Life
Victoria Boutenko

Gray's Anatomy
Henry Gray, F.R.S

Numbers and You
Lloyd Strayhorn

Power Healing
Dr. Zhi Gang Sha

Power vs. Force
David R. Hawkins, Ph. D.

The Complete Idiots Guide to Numerology
Kay Lagerquist, Ph. D., and Lisa Lenard

The Tao of Sexology
Dr. Stephen T. Chang

10 Essential Herbs
Lalitha Thomas

Any Anatomy Book

HEALTHY

TRANSITIONS

JOURNAL

This is a guide for the creation of your own Healthy Transitions Journal. You must purchase a journal and fill the pages accordingly.

Introduce yourself: (brief background statement.)

State your goals. Sum them up in a one-phrase statement. This will become your mantra.

Examples: I will be healthier than ever with each passing day. I am my own savior and keeper.

Using I will, exercises and strengthens your will. Using I am, speaks it into being.

Write down current physical condition and any present challenges. When doing this use language that renders the challenges powerless.

Examples: Up until now I was obese or overweight, but now I know I am simply over waste.
My anxiety and stress were causing issues in my physical body, but now that I can breathe they will subside.

Leave room in your journal either at the end of the day or week or whenever you see fit for Reflections. In this segment write down a personal note explaining how you feel about your transitions, where you came from, or what you are overcoming, and where you see yourself going. This can be a few short sentences or a paragraph or page or two, what ever is appropriate at the moment.

Take Inventory: Do this at the beginning and for stats that change every 1 to 2 weeks. Use the Weekly Progress Report. Here you can include other statistics that are relevant, blood sugar level, cholesterol, and so on.

Age:	Sex:
Height:	Weight:
Neck:	Face:
Upper Arm:	Wrist:
Chest/Bust:	Waste Line:
Hips:	Thighs:
Calves:	Ankles:
Blood Pressure:	Heart Rate (Pulse):
Breaths Per Minute:	BMI:
Vision:	

Describe food intake at present or over the last month. Use the Food and Activity Diary.

An easy way to do this is to save grocery and restaurant receipts. Be sure to include snacks, regular and irregular.

Describe typical weekday and weekend breakfast, lunch, dinner, and snacks.

Mon:

Tue:

Wed:

Thu:

Fri:

Sat:

Sun:

* As you transition continue to keep receipts. Make daily entries in journal on food intake.*

A word on grocery shopping, if you don't buy it and bring it into the house it won't go into your mouth or body; or those of other members of the household.

Describe typical exercise week before beginning healthy transition. Be as detailed as possible

Example:

Mon:	Walked 2 laps
Tue:	None
Wed:	Went to gym 20 min cardio
Thu:	Yoga 30 min
Fri:	3 push ups, walked 2 blocks, 4 squats, 2 sit-ups
Sat:	Walked around shopping mall 3 hrs
Sun:	Rested

As you transition write in journal daily exercises completed.

Example:

Mon: Breath of Life Clinic 7am, 12pm, 5pm, walked 4 laps
          7:15am, 10 Knee-Raises seated each leg 7:05am, 5:30pm
          Breath Mastery Technique (BMT), in car on way to and
          from work before getting out of or into bed.

Tue.

Wed:

Thu:

Fri:

Sat:

Sun:

* Remember to start small or slow and build, increasing as your
body adjusts to the new activity. *

Whenever you become comfortable, share your journal with those
who witness and share in your transitional journey. Then share with
those who need to see that they are not alone in their struggle, i.e. the
rest of the world.

If you are doing this with family, friends or co-workers encourage
all to write a journal. And while doing this set up sessions when you all
can share. Make this easy, regular but not mandatory. This exercise will
build support for all, and create a culture toward health and a healthy
community.

* In this transition develop language that Inner-gizes you, and Ex-
presses things that you don't need to hold on to. *

WEEKLY PROGRESS REPORT

WEEKLY	Wght	Chest	Arms	Waste	Thighs	BP	BPM	BMI
PROGRESS			L/R	Area	L/R			
WK 1 / /								
WK 2 / /								
WK 3 / /								
WK 4 / /								
WK 5 / /								
WK 6 / /								
WK 7 / /								
WK 8 / /								
WK 9 / /								
WK 10 / /								
WK 11 / /								
WK 12 / /								

12 Week Progress Chart. Chart measurements, Blood Pressure (BP), Breaths Per Minute (BPM), and Body Mass Index (BMI). Optimal number of Breaths is said to be 8. BMI calculator can be found online.

FOOD AND ACTIVITY CHART

Mo. Wk:	Food and Activity	Exercise Duration & Type	Dietary Supplement
Monday			
Tuesday			
Wednesday			
Thursday			
Friday			
Saturday			
Sunday			

ABOUT THE AUTHOR

Mottley, Aaron (Aration) Keith
11, 22, 33, 8

The numbers shown are the numerological translation of the name. Double-digits numbers are considered Master Numbers. 11 represents mastery of the principles of the number 1. Having a Master Number in the name or birth date means having a particular kind of potential and special purpose. Having one Master Number in your numerology is not uncommon. It is unusual to have more than one. Master Numbers indicate a cosmic contract to learn to master the potential of the given number and to teach and work to move humanity to a higher vibration. To operate on a Master Number level one must utilize cosmic, spiritual, universal, philosophical, or metaphysical principles. The authors explanation of the word COSMIC is Celestial Omniscient Spirit Manifesting In Consciousness. Each Master Number gives great potential around a specific energetic purpose. 11 represents the Spiritual Messenger. 22 represents the Master Builder. 33 represents the Master of Healing Energies Through Love. 8 represents leadership, personal power and prosperity. He is his mother's 7th born, 7 represents inner wisdom. This name comes a great deal of responsibility, which can be both challenging and gratifying. Realization has been tempered with acceptance, any potential power with humility. In his own words: "My innermost desire follows everything that the numbers have described. I will to help humanity gain principled awareness on a very basic level so that all can have the opportunity to achieve Mastery."

Master Barber / Barber Science Teacher

Herbalist

Biodynamic Nutritionist

Certified Holistic Health Consultant

Certified Kemetic Yoga Instructor

Breath Mastery Coach

Internal Fitness Trainer

INDEX

Web Addresses:
internalfitnesstrainer.com
inernalfitnesstrainer.wordpres
s.com